Stedman's

OB-GYN WORDS

STEDMANS

WILLIAMS & WILKINS
BALTIMORE • HONG KONG • LONDON • MUNICH
PHILADELPHIA • SYDNEY • TOKYO

Series Editor: Elizabeth Randolph
Editor: Maria Coughlin
Database Manager: Harriet Felscher
Production Manager: Cordelia Slaughter
Cover Design: Carla Frank

Williams & Wilkins
428 East Preston Street
Baltimore, Maryland 21202, USA

Printed in the United States of America

Library of Congress Cataloging-in-Publication Data

Stedman's OB-GYN words.
p. cm.
Developed from the database of Stedman's medical dictionary, 25th ed. and supplemented by terminology found in the current medical literature.
ISBN 0-683-07942-5
1. Gynecology—Dictionaries. 2. Obstetrics—Dictionaries. I. Stedman, Thomas Lathrop, 1853–1938. Medical dictionary.
[DNLM: 1. Gynecology—dictionaries. 2. Obstetrics—dictionaries.
WQ 13 S8124]
RG45.S74 1992
618′.014—dc20
DNLM/DLC
for Library of Congress

92-5543
CIP

92 93 94 95 96
1 2 3 4 5 6 7 8 9 10

Contents

ISBN: 0-683-079425 $28.00 + 6.66 S+H = $34.66

Barbara E Swanson
2400 41st St NW #106
Washington DC 20007-4911
202/965-7905

Result of Pap Test	What Result Means	Likely Next Step
Normal (no abnormal cells seen)	No abnormal cells	Pap test in 1 to 3 years, depending on age and other factors
ASC-US (atypical squamous cells of undetermined significance)	Cells look unusual but don't look exactly like dysplasia (75% of women with an ASC-US result have no abnormal cervical cells, but to be safe all women need additional testing or evaluation)	One of the following: ■ HPV test; if this is positive, then colposcopy; if negative, then Pap test in 1 year ■ Pap test in 4 to 6 months ■ Colposcopy
LSIL (Low-grade squamous intra-epithelial lesions)	Mildly abnormal cells (most women with a LSIL result have HPV infection, which will usually go away on its own, but to be safe all women need additional evaluation)	Colposcopy
HSIL (High-grade squamous intra-epithelial lesions)	Moderately to severely abnormal cells (all women need further evaluation)	Colposcopy

www.arhp.org/healthmatters

Acknowledgments

An important part of our editorial process is the involvement of medical transcriptionists—as advisors, reviewers, and/or editors. Special thanks go to the members of the Williams & Wilkins MT Advisory Board, whose expertise, ideas, and words contribute to the overall quality of this and other Stedman's word books: LaVonne Alexis, CMT; Joan Bachman; Addie M. Garner; Suzanne Minnick; Susan Pierce, CMT, ART; Laurie Spangler; Harriet Stewart; and Dorothy Vickers.

Explanatory Notes

Stedman's OB-GYN Words offers an authoritative assurance of quality and exactness to the wordsmiths of the health care professions—medical transcriptionists, medical editors and copy editors, medical records personnel and the many other users and producers of medical documentation. It can be used to validate both the spelling and accuracy of terminology in obstetrics and gynecology. This compilation of over 23,000 entries, fully cross-indexed for quick access, was built from a base vocabulary of 16,500 medical words, phrases, abbreviations and acronyms. This extensive A-Z list was developed from the database of *Stedman's Medical Dictionary 25ed.*, and supplemented by terminology found in the current medical literature.

Stedman's OB-GYN Words includes up-to-date terminology of obstetrics, gynecology and gynecologic oncology, maternal-fetal medicine, endocrinology, and infertility. The user will find listed here thousands of diseases and syndromes, traditional and new operative procedures and techniques (including colposcopy, laparoscopy, hysterosalpingography), diagnostic ultrasound terms, medications, lab test names, equipment and instrument names. Appendices of commonly performed OB-GYN procedures and related equipment terminology are featured at the back of the book. See Appendix 5 for illustrated fetal presentations.

Alphabetical Organization

Alphabetization of entries is letter by letter as spelled, ignoring punctuation, spaces, prefixed numbers, Greek letters, or other characters. For example:

acid-fast staining methods
acid formaldehyde hematin
α_1-acid glycoprotein
acid hematin

In subentries, the abbreviated singular form or the spelled-out plural form of the main entry word is ignored in alphabetization.

Format and Style

All main entries are in **boldface** to speed up location of a sought-after entry, to enhance distinction between main entries and sub-entries, and to relieve the textual density of the pages.

Irregular plurals and variant spellings are shown on the same line as the singular or preferred form of the word. For example:

villus, pl. villi
dilation, dilatation

Possessive forms that occur in the medical literature are retained in this reference. To form the non-possessives advocated by the American Association for Medical Transcription and other groups, simply drop the apostrophe or apostrophe "s" from the end of the word.

Cross-indexing

The A-Z word list is in an index-like main entry-subentry format that contains two combined alphabetical listings:

(1) A noun main entry-subentry organization typical of the A-Z section of medical dictionaries like *Stedman's*:

maneuver
- Bill's m.
- Bracht m.
- Brandt-Andrews m.
- Crede's m.

delivery
- abdominal d.
- assisted cephalic d.
- breech d.
- cesarean d.

(2) An adjective main entry-subentry organization, which lists words and phrases as you hear them. The main entries are the adjectives or modifiers in a multi-word term. The sub-entries are the nouns around which the terms are constructed and to which the adjectives or modifers pertain:

mammary
m. calculus
m. duct ectasia
m. dysplasia
m. fistula

endometrial
e. ablation
e. adenoacanthoma
e. adenosquamous carcinoma
e. atrophy

This format provides the user with more than one way to locate and identify a multi-word term. For example:

estrogen
catechol e.

catechol
c. estrogen

forceps
Halsted mosquito f.

Halsted
H. mosquito forceps

It also allows the user to see together all terms that contain a particular descriptor as well as all types, kinds, or variations of a noun entity. For example:

hydrops
fetal h., h. fetalis
h. folliculi
immune fetal h.
maternal h.

gonadotropin, gonadotrophin
chorionic g. (CG)
exogenous g.
g. pulsatile release
g. regulation

References

Stedman's medical dictionary. 25th ed. Baltimore: Williams & Wilkins, 1990.

Cunningham. Williams' obstetrics. 18th ed. East Norwalk, NJ: Appleton & Lange, 1989.

Herbst et al. Comprehensive gynecology. 2nd ed. St. Louis: Mosby Yearbook, 1992.

Creasy-Resnick. Maternal-fetal medicine. 2nd ed. Philadelphia: WB Saunders, 1989.

Cherry. Complications of pregnancy. 4th ed. Baltimore: Williams & Wilkins, 1991.

Gelehrter. Principles of medical genetics. Baltimore: Williams & Wilkins, 1990.

Jones. Novak's textbook of gynecology. 11th ed. Baltimore: Williams & Wilkins, 1988.

Briggs. Drugs in pregnancy and lactation. 3rd ed. Baltimore: Williams & Wilkins, 1990.

Berek. Practical gynecologic oncology. Baltimore: Williams & Wilkins, 1989.

Disaia. Clinical gynecologic oncology. 3rd ed. St. Louis: CV Mosby, 1989.

Speroff. Clinical gynecologic endocrinology and infertility. 4th ed. Baltimore: Williams & Wilkins, 1988.

Obstetrical & gynecological survey. Baltimore: Williams & Wilkins, 1991.

Contemporary Ob/Gyn. Montvale, NJ: Medical Economics, 1991.

Your Medical Word Resource Publisher

We strive to provide you with the most up-to-date and accurate word references available. Your use of this word book will prompt new editions, which will be published as often as justified by updates and revisions. We welcome your suggestions for improvements, changes, corrections, and additions—whatever will make this **Stedman's** product more useful to you. Please use the postpaid card at the back of this book and send your recommendations to the Reference Division at Williams & Wilkins.

A

Aase syndrome
Abbokinase
abdomen
fetal a.
pendulous a.
abdominal
a. approach
a. auscultation
a. circumference
a. delivery
a. distention
a. ectopic pregnancy
a. enlargement
a. examination
a. hernia
a. hysterectomy
a. hysteropexy
a. hysterotomy
a. incision
a. irradiation
a. myomectomy
a. pain
a. percussion
a. pregnancy
a. rescue
a. roentgenography
a. sacropexy
a. salpingectomy
a. salpingo-oophorectomy
a. salpingotomy
a. stria
a. strip radiotherapy
a. wall
a. wound
abdominocyesis
abdominohysterectomy
abdominohysterotomy
abdominopelvic
a. irradiation
a. scan
abdominovaginal hysterectomy
aberrant
abetalipoproteinemia
ablactation
ablation
endometrial a.
laser a.
Nd-YAG laser a.
ablatio placentae
abnormal
a. cortisol secretion
a. embryo
a. feedback signals
a. fetal behavior
a. fetal development
a. hysterosalpingography
a. infant
a. labor
a. menstruation
a. pregnancy
a. response
a. transformation zone
a. uterine bleeding
abnormality
central nervous system a.
cervical a.
chromosomal a.
chromosomal structural a.
congenital a.
cord a.
deflexion a.
disk a.
fetal a.
fetal abdominal a.
fetal postural a.
fetal thoracic a.
fibrinogen a.
genetic a.
genitourinary a.
gestational a.
hand a.
hand bone a.
hormone a.
lumbosacral intervertebral disk a.
müllerian a.
neurologic a.
nonpalpable a.
ovarian a.
reproductive tract a.
sex chromosomal a.
skeletal a.
soft tissue a.
urinary tract a.
uterine a.
vaginal epithelial a.
X-chromosome a.
ABO
ABO antigen

ABO *(continued)*
ABO blood group system
ABO hemolytic disease of the newborn
ABO incompatibility
abort
aborted ectopic pregnancy
abortient
abortifacient
abortigenic
abortion
accidental a.
ampullar a.
aneuploid a.
complete a.
criminal a.
euploid a.
habitual a.
imminent a.
incipient a.
incomplete a.
induced a.
inevitable a.
infected a.
justifiable a.
menstrual extraction a.
missed a.
a. rate
recurrent a.
recurrent spontaneous a.
repeated a.
second trimester a.
selective a.
septic a.
spontaneous a.
surgically induced a.
therapeutic a.
threatened a.
tubal a.
abortionist
abortive
abortus
abruption
placental a.
abruptio placentae
abscess
Bartholin's a.
ovarian a.
parametric a.
parametritic a.
pelvic a.
perinephric a.
premammary a.
tubo-ovarian a.
absence
uterine a.
vaginal a.
absolute sterility
absorbable
a. gelatin sponge
a. staple
a. suture
absorptiometry
dual-energy x-ray a. (DEXA)
single-photon a.
absorption
calcium a.
a. fever
fluorescent treponemal antibody a. (FTA-ABS)
abstinence
abuse
alcohol a.
child a.
maternal cocaine a.
maternal drug a.
sexual a.
acanthosis nigricans
accelerated starvation
accelerator
linear a.
access
fetoplacental a.
uterine a.
accessory
a. breast
a. nipple
a. ovary
a. placenta
accident
cerebrovascular a. (CVA)
obstetrical a.
accidental
a. abortion
a. fetal injury
a. hemorrhage
a. pregnancy
accompanying mood state
accouchement
a. forcé
accoucheur
accretion
bone a.

accuracy
assay a.
diagnostic a.
Accurbron
Accutane
acebutolol
acenocoumarin
acenocoumarol
Aceta
acetaminophen
acetate
cyproterone a.
demedroxyprogesterone a. (DMPA)
flecainide a.
leuprolide a.
medroxyprogesterone a. (MPA)
megestrol a.
nafarelin a.
norethindrone a.
quingestanol a.
acetazolamide
acetic acid
acetohexamide
acetone
acetonide
fluocinolone a.
triamcinolone a.
acetonuria
acetophenazine
acetophenetidin
acetophenide
dihydroxyprogesterone a.
aceto-white epithelium
acetoxyprogesterone derivative
acetylcholine
acetylcholinesterase (AchE)
acetyldigitoxin
acetylsalicylic acid
a-chain of ricin
achalasia
AchE
acetylcholinesterase
achievement
pregnancy a.
achondroplasia
achordia
Achromycin
acid
acetic a.
acetylsalicylic a.
amino a.
D-amino a.
L-amino a.
aminocaproic a.
arachidonic a.
arylalkanoic a.
arylcarboxylic a.
arylpropionic a.
ascorbic a.
a. aspiration syndrome
bile a.
boric a.
carbonic a.
clavulanic a.
deoxyadenylic a. (dAMP)
deoxycytidylic a. (dCMP)
deoxyguanylic a. (dGMP)
deoxyribonucleic a. (DNA)
deoxythymidylic a. (dTMP)
epsilon-aminocaproic a., ε-aminocaproic a. (EACA)
ethacrynic a.
flufenamic a.
folic a.
folinic a.
free fatty a.
fusanic a.
hydriodic a.
5-hydroxyindoleacetic a. (5-HIAA)
iocetamic a.
iopanoic a.
linoleic a.
lysergic a.
mandelic a.
mefenamic a.
messenger ribonucleic a.
nalidixic a.
nicotinic a.
noncarbonic a.
nonvolatile a.
pantothenic a.
para-aminomethylbenzoic a. (PAMBA)
para-aminosalicylic a.
a. phosphatase
retinoic a.
ribonucleic a. (RNA)
salicylsalicylic a.
sialic a.
sodium citrate with citric a.
tolfenamic a.
tranexamic a.

acid *(continued)*
transfer ribonucleic a. (tRNA)
trichloroacetic a.
2,4,5-trichlorophenoxyacetic a.
uric a.
valproic a.
volatile a.
acid-base
a.-b. balance
a.-b. equilibrium
a.-b. measurement
a.-b. state
a.-b. status
a.-b. value
acidemia
argininosuccinic a.
fetal a.
metabolic a.
methylmalonic a.
mixed umbilical arterial a.
pyroglutamic a.
acidic fibroblast growth factor (FGFa)
acidosis
fetal a.
lactic a.
metabolic a.
perinatal a.
respiratory a.
aciduria
hereditary orotic a.
methylmalonic a.
acne
a. drug
a. vulgaris
acoustic stimulation study
acquired
a. hemolytic anemia
a. immunodeficiency syndrome (AIDS)
a. immunodeficiency syndrome-related virus (ARV)
acrochordon
acrocyanosis
acromegaly
acromion presentation
acrosin
acrosome
a. reaction
Act
Model Uniform Parentage A.
Actamin
act-FU-Cy
actinomycin D, 5-fluorouracil, cyclophosphamide
ACTH
adrenocorticotropic hormone
ACTH stimulation test
Acthar
Actidil
actin
actin-myosin interaction
Actinomyces
A. israelii
A. urinary tract infection
actinomycin D
actinomycin D, 5-fluorouracil, cyclophosphamide (act-FU-Cy)
actinomycosis
action
fetal heart a.
gene a.
law of mass a.
luteolytic a.
mediating a.
self-priming a.
uterine a.
activated partial thromboplastin time (APTT)
activation
activator
lymphocyte a.
plasminogen a. (PA)
urokinase-type plasminogen a. (u-PA)
active
a. phase
a. third-stage management
activin
activity
antigen a.
elevated enzyme a.
endometrial cycling a.
enzyme a.
fetal a.
lupus anticoagulant a.
lymphotoxin antitumor a.
mitogenic a.
opioid a.
ovarian a.
peripheral androgen a.

phospholipase a.
sexual a.
uterine a.
actuarial survival
acuminata
a. condylomata
acupuncture
acute
a. anaphylaxis
a. fatty liver
a. iliofemoral venous thrombectomy
a. intermittent porphyria
a. interstitial pneumonia
a. pelvic pain
a. pyelonephritis
a. renal failure
a. salpingitis
a. tubular necrosis
a. urethral syndrome
acyclic pelvic pain
acyclovir
Adalat
Adapin
adaptation
maternal ocular a.
ADC
AIDS dementia complex
addiction
alcohol a.
cocaine a.
drug a.
opioid a.
addisonian
a. crisis
a. pernicious anemia
Addison's disease
adenine
a. arabinoside
adenitis
sclerosing a.
vestibular a.
adenoacanthoma
endometrial a.
lymph node endometriotic a.
adenocarcinoma
cervical clear cell a.
clear cell a.
endometrial a.
endometrial clear cell a.
endometrial secretory a.
mesonephric a.
metastatic a.
ovarian clear cell a.
papillary a.
serous a.
a. of uterus
vaginal a.
vaginal clear cell a.
vulvar adenoid cystic a.
adenofibroma
adenofibromyoma
adenofibrosis
adenohypophysis
adenohypophysitis
lymphocytic a.
adenoid cystic carcinoma
adenoleiomyofibroma
adenoma
apocrine a.
a. of breast
ductal a.
growth hormone-secreting a.
lactating a.
a. malignum
a. of nipple
ovarian tubular a.
parathyroid a.
pituitary a.
prolactin-secreting a.
suspected pituitary a.
testosterone-secreting adrenal a.
virilizing a.
adenomatoid
a. oviduct tumor
a. tumor
adenomatosis
erosive a. of nipple
fibrosing a.
adenomatous
a. endometrial hyperplasia
a. hyperplasia
a. polyp
adenomyoma
adenomyosis
a. uteri
a. in uterine enlargement
adenopathy
axillary a.
postinflammatory a.
adenosalpingitis
adenosarcoma
müllerian a.

adenosine
a. 3′,5′-cyclic monophosphate
a. deaminase
a. monophosphate (AMP)
a. phosphate
a. triphosphate (ATP)
a. triphosphate (ATP)
adenosis
blunt duct a.
fibrosing a.
microglandular a.
sclerosing a.
vaginal a.
adenosquamous
a. carcinoma
a. endometrial carcinoma
adenylate cyclase
adenyl cyclase
adherent placenta
adhesion
amniotic a.'s
intrauterine a.
a. lysis
peritubal a.
platelet a.
a. prevention
adhesive
a. disease
a. vaginitis
a. vulvitis
Adipex-P
adipocere
adipose tissue
adjustment
psychosocial a.
adjuvant
a. chemotherapy
Freund's a.
a. radiotherapy
a. therapy
administration
bicarbonate a.
immunoglobulin a.
oral a.
pulsatile GnRH a.
sequential a.
transdermal a.
vaginal a.
admission order
admittance procedure
adnexal
a. cyst
a. infection
a. mass
a. metastasis
a. torsion
a. tumor
adnexectomy
adnexitis
adnexopexy
adnexum, pl. **adnexa**
adolescence
adolescent
a. breast
a. gynecology
a. pregnancy
a. sterility
adoption
adoptive immunotherapy
adrenal
a. androgen
a. crisis
a. gland
a. gland disease
a. gland morphology
a. hyperandrogenism
a. hyperandrogenism marker
a. hyperplasia
a. insufficiency
Marchand's a.'s
a. morphologic consideration
a. neoplasm
a. rest tumor
a. steroid
a. tumor
a. virilism
a. virilizing syndrome
adrenalectomy
Adrenalin
adrenaline injection
adrenarche
premature a.
adrenergic
a. blocker
a. drug
a. receptor
a. stimulator
α-adrenergic
β-adrenergic
β-a. agent
β-a. agonist
adrenocortical
a. function
a. hormone
a. insufficiency

a. steroid
a. steroidogenesis
adrenocorticotropic hormone (ACTH)
adrenocorticotropin
chorionic a.
adrenogenital syndrome
adrenoleukodystrophy
Adriamycin
Adson
A. forceps
A. ganglion scissors
A. pick-ups
Adsorbocarpine
adult
a. ovary
a. respiratory distress syndrome (ARDS)
adult-onset congenital adrenal hyperplasia
advanced
a. abdominal pregnancy
a. ovarian carcinoma
a. vulvar carcinoma
adverse outcome
adynamic ileus
aerobe
aerobic metabolism
aerocolpos
Aerolate
Aerolone
Aeroseb-Dex
afetal
affective disorder
affinity
afibrinogenemia
congenital a.
Afko-Lube
AFP
alpha-fetoprotein
Afrinol
afterbirth
agalactia
agalactorrhea
agalactosis
agalactous
age
childbearing a.
developmental a.
fertilization a.
fetal a.
gestational a.
growth-adjusted sonographic a. (GASA)
maternal a.
menstrual a.
ovulation a.
ovulatory a.
paternal a.
postconception a.
agency
state health a.
agenesis
gonadal a.
müllerian a.
renal a.
vaginal a.
agent
β-adrenergic a.
alkylating a.
anticancer a.
antifibrinolytic a.
antifolic a.
antineoplastic a.
antiplatelet a.
antiprostaglandin a.
beta-adrenergic a.
$beta_2$-adrenergic a.
chemotherapeutic a.
cosmetic a.
cycle-nonspecific a.
cycle-specific a.
cytotoxic a.
delta a.
fibrinolytic a.
hyperosmotic a.
infertility a.
myelosuppressive a.
nonalkylating a.
oncogenic a.
pressor a.
progestational a.
sclerosing a.
teratogenic a.
tocolytic a.
Agent Orange
agglutination
labial a.
latex a.
a. test
agglutinin
aggregation
platelet a.
aggressive treatment

Aging
Select Committee on A.
aging gamete
agitated depression
agonadism
agonist
beta-adrenergic a.
calcium a.
cholinergic a.
dopamine a.
dopamine receptor a.
dopaminergic a.
gonadotropin-releasing hormone a.
β-receptor a.
agranulocytosis
A/G ratio
albumin/globulin ratio
Ahumada-Del Castillo syndrome
AID
artificial insemination donor
AIDS
acquired immunodeficiency syndrome
AIDS dementia complex (ADC)
AIDS-related complex (ARC)
AIH
artificial insemination by husband
AIHA
autoimmune hemolytic anemia
air leak syndrome
airway
a. conductance
a. resistance
a. suction
AJCC
American Joint Committee for Cancer Staging
Akineton
alanine aminotransferase
albinism
albumin
plasma a.
serum a.
albumin/globulin ratio (A/G ratio, A/G ratio)
albuminuria
albuterol
Alcock's canal
alcohol
a. abuse
a. addiction
a. ingestion
nicotinyl a.
alcoholism
maternal a.
Alconefrin
Aldactone
Aldomet
Aldoril
aldosterone
aldosteronism
Aldridge sling procedure
alimentation
intravenous a.
parenteral a.
Alka-Butazolidin
alkalemia
alkaline phosphatase
alkaloid
levorotatory a.
plant a.
Veratrum a.
Vinca a.
alkalosis
respiratory a.
alkaptonuria
Alka-Seltzer
Alkeran
alkylating
a. agent
a. chemotherapy
allantoic cyst
allantoidoangiopagous twins
allantoidoangiopagus
allantois
allele
Allen-Masters syndrome
Allerest nasal
allergen
allergy
sperm a.
alligator forceps
alligator-jaw instrument
Allis
A. clamp
A. forceps
all or none phenomenon
alloantibody
alloantigen
allogeneic
a. disease
a. fetal graft
allogenicity

allograft
a. survival
alloimmune
a. factor
a. mechanism
a. neonatal thrombocytopenic purpura
a. thrombocytopenia
alloimmunity
alloimmunization
allowance
recommended dietary a.
alopecia
alpha
a. error
a. interferon
a. particle
transforming growth factor a. (TGFα)
17alpha-acetoxyprogesterone derivative
alpha-adrenergic, α-adrenergic
a.-a. blocker
a.-a. receptor
a.-a. stimulator
alpha-1-antitrypsin
Alphaderm
17-alpha-ethinyl testosterone
alpha-fetoprotein, α-fetoprotein (AFP)
amniotic fluid a.-f.
a.-f. elevation
a.-f. level
maternal serum a.-f. (MSAFP)
alpha-melanotrophin
Alphamine
alphaprodine
alpha-recombinant interferon
alpha-1 thymosin product
alprazolam
alteration
uterine activity a.
aludrine
Alupent
Alurate
alveolus, pl. **alveoli**
amantadine
amastia
amaurosis
amazia
ambenonium
ambiguity
genital a.
sexual a.
ambiguous genitalia
amboceptor
ambulation
early a.
ambulatory
a. care
a. uterine contraction testing
Amcill
amebiasis
amebic vaginitis
Amen
amenia
amenorrhea
athletic a.
dietary a.
emotional a.
eugonadotropic a.
hypergonadotropic a.
hyperprolactinemic a.
hypogonadotropic a.
hypophysial a.
hypothalamic a.
jogger's a.
lactation a.
ovarian a.
pathologic a.
physiologic a.
postmenopausal a.
postpartum a.
postpill a.
primary a.
secondary a.
traumatic a.
amenorrhea-galactorrhea syndrome
amenorrheal, amenorrheic
American
A. Cancer Society
A. Cancer Society mammography recommendations
A. College of Obstetricians and Gynecologists
A. Fertility Society
A. Fertility Society classification of endometriosis
A. Joint Committee for Cancer Staging (AJCC)

American *(continued)*
A. Joint Committee for Cancer Staging and End Results Reporting
A. Society of Anesthesiologists
amethopterin
ametria
Amfetamine
Amicar
amikacin
Amikin
amiloride
amino
a. acid
a. acid metabolism
D-amino acid
L-amino acid
aminoaciduria
aminocaproic acid
aminoglutethimide
aminoglycoside
aminopeptidase
leucine a.
aminophylline
aminoprine
aminopterin
aminopyrine
amino-terminal peptide
aminotransferase
alanine a.
aspartate a.
amiodarone
Amipaque
Amitid
Amitril
amitriptyline
ammoniac
sal a.
ammonium
a. bromide
a. chloride
amnestic response
amniocentesis
genetic a.
amniochorion
amniography
a. in hydatidiform mole
amniohook
amnioinfusion
amnioma
amnion
a. nodosum
a. ring
a. rupture
amnionic
a. caruncle
a. fluid
amnionitis
silent a.
amniorrhea
amniorrhexis
amnioscope
amnioscopy
amniostat-FLM
amniotic
a. adhesions
a. band anomalad
a. bands
a. cavity
a. cavity bacterial infection
a. fluid
a. fluid alpha-fetoprotein
a. fluid cell culture
a. fluid embolism
a. fluid level
a. fluid pocket
a. fluid quantitation
a. fluid syndrome
a. sac
a. sheet
amniotome
amniotomy
amobarbital
A-mode ultrasound
amotio placentae
amoxapine
amoxicillin
Amoxil
AMP
adenosine monophosphate
amphetamine
amphotericin B
ampicillin
amplification
DNA a.
Y-specific DNA a.
ampulla of oviduct
ampullar
a. abortion
a. pregnancy
amputation
birth a.
cervical a.
congenital a.

intrauterine a.
spontaneous a.
Amrinone
Amsacrine (mAMSA)
amygdalin
amylase
serum a.
amylase-creatinine clearance ratio
amyl nitrite
amylobarbitone
amylophagia
Amytal
anacatadidymus
anadidymus
anaerobe
Anafranil
anagen
anal
a. canal
a. incontinence
a. sphincter disruption
analgesia
caudal a.
conduction a.
continuous epidural a.
epidural a.
narcotic a.
peridural a.
perineal a.
regional a.
spinal a.
analgesic
narcotic a.
analogue
gonadotropin-releasing hormone a.
luteinizing hormone-releasing hormone a.
oxytocin a.
tetracycline a.
analysis
automated multiple a.
blood a.
cell block a.
chromosomal a.
clinicopathological a.
linkage a.
molecular a.
molecular genetic a.
multivariate a.
postoperative symptom a.
preoperative symptom a.
saturation a.
semen a.
anamnestic response
anaphase
a. lag
anaphylaxis
acute a.
recurrent a.
anaplastic carcinoma
Anaprox
anasarca
fetoplacental a.
Anaspaz
anastomosis, pl. **anastomoses**
colorectal a.
cornual a.
microsurgical tubocornual a.
ureterotubal a.
ureteroureteral a.
anatomic rigidity
anatomy
fetal a.
fetal intracranial a.
immune system a.
intracranial a.
Ancef
Ancobon
Ancotil
androblastoma
androgen
adrenal a.
a. antagonist
a. dynamics
excess a.
a. excess
a. insensitivity
a. insensitivity syndrome
a. interaction
a. receptor
a. resistance
a. secretion
androgenesis
androgenized woman
androgenous
androgen-producing tumor
android
a. obesity
a. pelvis
androstane
3α-androstanediol glucuronide
5α-androstane-3α,17β-diol glucuronide (3α-diol-G)
androstenedione

androsterone
a. glucuronide
anechoic tissue
anectasis
anembryonic gestation
anemia
acquired hemolytic a.
addisonian pernicious a.
angiopathic hemolytic a.
aplastic a.
autoimmune acquired hemolytic a.
autoimmune hemolytic a. (AIHA)
congenital a.
Cooley's a.
Fanconi's a.
hemolytic a.
hereditary nonspherocytic a.
hypoplastic a.
iron deficiency a.
macrocytic a. of pregnancy
megaloblastic a.
pernicious a.
pregnancy-associated hypoplastic a.
sickle cell a.
anemic effect
anencephalic newborn
anencephaly
anergy
Anestacon
anesthesia
caudal a.
conduction a.
epidural a.
extradural a.
general a.
inhalation a.
inhalational a.
local a.
lumbar epidural a.
maternal a.
obstetric a.
paracervical a.
peridural a.
perineal a.
pudendal a.
regional a.
saddle block a.
spinal a.
anesthesiologist
a. consultation
anesthetic
gas a.
a. gas exposure
local a.
volatile a.
aneuploid abortion
aneuploidy
aneurysm
aortic a.
arterial a.
dissecting aortic a.
intracranial a.
ruptured cerebral a.
saccular a.
angel dust
angina
angiogenesis
angiogenic growth factor
angiography
pulmonary a.
angiokeratoma
vulvar a.
angiolysis
angioma
cerebral a.
dural spinal a.
intradural spinal a.
spider a.
spinal a.
angiomatoid tumor
angiomyoma of oviduct
angiopathic hemolytic anemia
angiosarcoma
uterine a.
angiotensin
angiotensin II
angiotensinogen
angle
urethral a.
urethrovesical a.
anhedonia
Anhydron
ani
levator a.
anileridine
aniridia
anisindione
anisomastia
anisotropine
ankylocolpos
ankylosing spondylitis
anlage
annexectomy

annexitis
annexopexy
annual visit
annular
a. band
a. placenta
a. tubule
anogenital wart
anomalad
amniotic band a.
holoprosencephaly a.
Robin a.
anomalous uterus
anomaly
cardiac a.
cervical a.
chromosomal a.
congenital a.
Ebstein's a.
fetal a.
fetal vascular a.
genetic a.
intracranial dural vascular a.
müllerian a.
orthopaedic a.
sex chromosomal a.
umbilical cord a.
uterine a.
vaginal a.
vascular a.
anorchia
anorectic
a. reaction
Anorex
anorexia
anorexia nervosa
anosmia
anovular
a. menstruation
anovulation
persistent a.
anovulational menstruation
anovulatory
a. bleeding
a. infertility
a. patient
anoxia
a. neonatorum
Ansaid
Anspor
Antabuse
antacid
antagonism
antagonist
androgen a.
calcium a.
folic acid a.
follicle-stimulating hormone a.
gonadotropin-releasing hormone a.
narcotic a.
opioid receptor a.
antagonist-induced gonadotropin deprivation
antecedent
cerebral palsy a.
anteflex
anteflexion
antenatal
a. anti-D immunoglobulin
a. diagnosis
a. patient
a. phenobarbitol treatment
a. screening
a. ultrasound
antepartum
a. bleeding
a. care
a. hemorrhage
anteposition
anterior
a. asynclitism
a. exenteration
occiput a. (OA)
a. pelvic exenteration
a. pituitary-like hormone
a. urethritis
anteroposterior diameter
anteversion
anteverted
anthropoid pelvis
antibacterial therapy
antibiotic
beta-lactam a.
beta-lactamase-resistant antistaphylococcal a., β-lactamase-resistant antistaphylococcal a.
prophylactic a.
antibody
anticardiolipin a.
anti-HIV a.
anti-idiotype a.
anti-M a.

antibody *(continued)*
antinuclear a.
antipaternal antileukocytotoxic a.
antiphospholipid a.
antisperm a.
blood group a.
circulating platelet a.
cytophilic a.
hemagglutinating inhibition a. (HIA)
humoral a.
IgM a.
lupus anticoagulant a.
maternal a.
monoclonal a.
natural a.
ovarian a.
phospholipid a.
platelet-associated a.
polyclonal a.
a. reaction site
resistance to a.
a. response
a. screening
serum a.
sperm a.
anticancer agent
anticardiolipin
a. antibody
anticholinergic
a. drug
anticholinesterase
anticoagulant
lupus a.
a. therapy
anticoagulation
anticodon
anticonvulsant
anti-D
a.-D. gamma globulin
a.-D. immunoglobulin
antidepressant
a. therapy
tricyclic a.
antidiuretic hormone
antiembolism stocking
antiemetic therapy
antiestrogen
antiestrogenic effect
antiferritin antibody
antifibrinolytic agent
antifolic agent
antifungal drug
antigalactagogue
antigalactic
antigen
ABO a.
a. activity
a. binding site
CA-125 a.
carcinoembryonic a. (CEA)
cell surface a.
a. determinant
Forssman a.
hepatitis B surface a. (HBsAg)
heterophil a.
histocompatibility a.
histocompatibility locus a.
human leukocyte a. (HLA)
human lymphocyte a.
H-Y a.
incompatible blood group a.
M a.
major histocompatibility a.
nuclear a.
oncofetal a.
platelet a.
red cell a.
Rh a.
surface a.
thymic lymphocyte a. (TL)
a. tolerance
transplantation a.
tumor a.
tumor-associated a. (TAA)
tumor-specific transplantation a.
antigen-125
carcinoembryonic a.-125 (CEA-125)
carcinoma a.-125
antigen-antibody complex
antigenic
a. modulation
a. paralysis
antigenicity
tumor a.
antigen-sensitive cell
antiglobulin test
antigonadotropin
antihelminthic therapy
antihistamine
anti-HIV antibody

antihypertensive
a. drug
a. therapy
anti-idiotype antibody
antiluteogenic
antimalarial drug
anti-M antibody
antimetabolite
antimicrobial
beta-lactam a.
a. therapy
Antiminth
antineoplastic
a. agent
a. drug
antinuclear antibody
antiparasitic drug therapy
antipaternal antileukocytotoxic antibody
antiphospholipid
a. antibody
antiplatelet agent
Antipress
antiprogesterone
antiprogestin
antiprostaglandin
a. agent
a. treatment
antipsychotic drug
antipyretic
antireceptor
antishock trousers
antisialagogue
antispasmodic
antisperm antibody
antithrombin II
antithrombin III
antithymocyte globulin
antithyroid
a. drug
antitreponemal test
Anti-Tuss
antiviral therapy
antral follicle
anuria
anus, gen. and pl. **ani**
imperforate a.
vaginal ectopic a.
vestibular a.
vulvovaginal a.
anxiety
aorta, gen. and pl. **aortae**
coarctation of a.
descending a.
fetal a.
overriding a.
aortic
a. aneurysm
a. laceration
a. node
a. node metastasis
a. regurgitation
a. stenosis
a. valve disease
a. valve insufficiency
apareunia
Apgar score
aphtha, pl. **aphthae**
Bednar's aphthae
aplastic anemia
apnea
apocrine
a. adenoma
a. cyst
a. gland
a. miliaria
apolipoprotein
apoplexy
uteroplacental a.
apoprotein
apoprotein A
apoptosis
apparatus, pl. **apparatus**
Heyns' abdominal decompression a.
appearance
meconium ileus a.
appendectomy
appendicitis
appendix
application
topical iodine a.
applicator
Fletcher-Suit a.
approach
abdominal a.
transrectal a.
Apresoline
aprobarbital
aprotinin
APTT
activated partial thromboplastin time
Aquachloral
AquaMEPHYTON
Aquaphyllin

APGAR - Appearance, Pulse, Grimace, Activity, Respiratory

Aquasol A
Aquasol E
Aquatensen
aqueductal stenosis
arabinoside
adenine a.
cytosine a.
arabinosylcytosine
arachidonic
a. acid
arachnoiditis
Aralen
Aramine
arborization
arbor vitae
ARC
AIDS-related complex
arch
pubic a.
architectural disturbance
architecture
histologic a.
pelvic a.
arcuate
a. artery
a. ligament of pubis
a. nucleus
a. uterus
ARDS
adult respiratory distress syndrome
area
skip a.
areola, pl. **areolae**
a. umbilicus
areolar connective tissue
Arfonad
arginine
a. vasopressin
a. vasotocin
argininosuccinic acidemia
argininosuccinicaciduria
argon beam coagulator
Argonz-Del Castillo syndrome
Arias-Stella
A.-S. effect
A.-S. phenomenon
A.-S. reaction
Aristocort
Arlidin
arm
brawny a.
nuchal a.
Army-Navy retractor
aromatase
aromatization
arrest
cardiac a.
a. disorder
follicular development a.
preterm labor a.
arrhenoblastoma
arrhythmia
cardiac a.
fetal a.
Artane
arterenol
arterial
a. aneurysm
a. blood gas
a. blood pressure
a. calcification
a. linear density
a. occlusive disease
a. vascular bed
a. vascular disease
a. waveform
arteriogram
pelvic a.
arteriography
arteriosus
ductus a.
patent ductus a.
arteriovenous
a. malformation
a. oxygen difference
artery
arcuate a.
azygos a.
basal a.
carotid a.
cervical a.
circumflex a.
coiled a.
colic a.
deep circumflex iliac a.
endometrial spiral a.
epigastric a.
femoral circumflex a.
fetal cranial a.
hemorrhoidal a.
hypogastric a.
ileocolic a.
iliac a.
inferior mesenteric a.
lumbar a.

mesenteric a.
middle sacral a.
obturator a.
ovarian a.
pelvic a.
pudendal a.
radial a.
spiral a.
superior mesenteric a.
umbilical a.
uterine a.
vaginal a.
vertebral a.

arthritis
juvenile rheumatoid a.
psoriatic a.
rheumatoid a.

Arthritis Pain Formula

Arthropan

Arthus reaction

artifact
deodorant a.

artificial
a. insemination
a. insemination donor (AID)
a. insemination by husband (AIH)
a. pacemaker

ARV
acquired immunodeficiency syndrome-related virus

arylalkanoic acid

arylcarboxylic acid

arylpropionic acid

AS
Crysticillin AS
Duracillin AS
Pentids-P AS
Pfizerpen AS

ascensus

Aschheim-Zondek test (A.-Z. test)

ascites
tumor a.

ascorbic acid

Ascriptin

Ascriptin A/D

Asendin

Asepto syringe

Asherman's syndrome

Ashkenazi Jew

Asmalix

aspartate aminotransferase

aspect
medicolegal a.'s

Aspergum

asphyxia
birth a.
blue a.
fetal a.
a. livida
a. neonatorum
a. pallida
perinatal a.

aspiration
a. biopsy
cyst a.
fine-needle a.
gastric a.
a. of gastric contents
gastric fluid a.
meconium a.
menstrual a.
needle a.
a. pneumonitis
a. prevention
a. prophylaxis
vacuum a.

aspirator
Vabra a.
vacuum a.

aspirin

assault
sexual a.

assay
a. accuracy
biologic a.
CA-125 a.
enzyme a.
enzyme-linked immunosorbent a. (ELISA)
estradiol a.
hamster egg penetration a.
hormone a.
immunologic a.
immunoradiometric a. (IRMA)
limulus amebocyte lysate a.
a. marker
microhemagglutination a. (MHA)
radioreceptor a.
receptor a.
sandwich a.
a. sensitivity
a. specificity

assay *(continued)*
sperm penetration a.
stem cell a.
thyroid-stimulating hormone a.
tumor-cloning a.
assessment
high-risk pregnancy a.
historical a.
periodic patient a.
ultrasound a.
assignment
sex a.
assisted
a. cephalic delivery
a. conception
a. reproduction
associated dysfunction
association constant
asthenospermia
asthma
bronchial a.
maternal a.
AsthmaHaler
AsthmaNefrin
Astler-Coller modification of Dukes' classification
asymmetry
asymptomatic
a. bacteriuria
a. genital herpes
a. infection
a. infertility
a. maternal infection
a. mild endometriosis
a. myoma
a. newborn
a. viral shedding
asynclitism
anterior a.
posterior a.
Atabrine
Atarax
ataxia telangiectasia
atelectasis
primary a.
secondary a.
atenolol
atherosclerosis
atherosis
athlete
athletic amenorrhea
Ativan
atony
uterine a.
atopic dermatitis
atopy
ATP
adenosine triphosphate
atresia
choanal a.
esophageal a.
a. folliculi
vaginal a.
atretic
a. cervix
a. follicle
atrial
a. bigeminy
a. fibrillation
a. flutter
a. natriuretic peptide
a. septal defect
atrioventricular (AV)
a. block
a. septal defect
at-risk pregnancy
Atromid-S
atrophic
a. change
a. vaginitis
atrophy
endometrial a.
linear a.
postmenopausal a.
skin a.
traction a.
vaginal a.
atropine
attack
transient ischemic a. (TIA)
attenuating tissue
Attenuvax
attitude
fetal a.
maternal a.
postpartum a.
attrition
follicular a.
sperm a.
atypia
bowenoid a.
koilocytic a.
vulvar a.

atypical
a. epithelium
a. vessel colposcopic pattern
^{198}Au
gold-198
Auerbach's plexus
augmentation
labor a.
a. mammaplasty
oxytocin a.
augmented breast
Augmentin
Aureomycin
aurothioglucose
auscultation
abdominal a.
periodic a.
autoantibody
thyroid a.
typhoid a.
autoantigen
autochthonous tumor
autocrine
a. communication
autograft
autoimmune
a. acquired hemolytic anemia
a. disease
a. factor
a. hemolytic anemia (AIHA)
a. mechanism
a. oophoritis
a. thrombocytopenic purpura
autoimmunity
autoinoculation
autologous
a. blood
a. blood donation
a. bone marrow reinfusion
a. transfusion
automated multiple analysis
autonomic nervous system
autosite
autosomal
a. chromosome disorder
a. deletion
a. disorder
a. dominant disorder
a. dominant inheritance
a. dominant trait
a. monosomy
a. recessive disorder
a. recessive inheritance
a. recessive trait
a. trisomy
autotransfusion
Auvard speculum
AV
atrioventricular
Aventyl
average radiation dose
Avitene
axial resolution
axilla
axillary
a. adenopathy
a. hematoma
a. lymphadenopathy
a. lymph node
a. skin lesion
a. tail
a. tail of Spence
a. view
axis, pl. **axes**
conjugate a.
gonadal a.
hypothalamic-hypophyseal-ovarian-endometrial a.
hypothalamic-pituitary a.
hypothalamic-pituitary-gonadal a.
pelvic a.
a. pelvis
pituitary a.
a. traction
axis-traction forceps
Ayercillin
Ayers spatula
Azactam
azatadine
azathioprine
azidothymidine (AZT)
azoospermia
Azo-Standard
azotemia
prerenal a.
Azovan Blue
AZT
azidothymidine
A.-Z. test
aztreonam
azygos artery

B

B
B cell
B complex vitamins
B lymphocyte
Babcock clamp
babesiosis
Babson chart
baby
blue b.
blueberry muffin b.
giant b.
juice b.
test-tube b.
bacampicillin
Bacarate
Baciguent
Bacille bilié de Calmette-Guérin (BCG)
bacillus
b. Calmette-Guérin (BCG)
bacitracin
backache
Backhaus clamp
baclofen
bacteremia
polymicrobial b.
bacteria
b. count
bacterial
b. contamination
b. cystitis
b. endocarditis
b. growth
b. infection
b. recovery
b. toxin
b. vaginosis
bacteriology
bacteriuria
asymptomatic b.
Bacteroides
B. fragilis
Bactocill
Bactrim
bag
b. of waters
balance
acid-base b.
fetal acid-base b.
sodium b.
transcapillary fluid b.
balanced
b. chromosomal inversion
b. translocation
balanitis
b. circinata
b. circumscripta plasmacellularis
plasma cell b.
b. of Zoon
Baldy's operation
Balfour
B. bladder blade
B. retractor
Ballard chart
Ballentine clamp
balloon catheter technique
ballottable
ballottement
Balminil
band
amniotic b.'s
annular b.
C b.
G b.
Q b.
R b.
T b.
bandage scissors
banding
chromosomal b.
b. pattern
Bandl
pathologic retraction ring of B.
Bandl's ring
Banthine
barbiturate
bariatric surgery
barium
b. enema
b. study
barium-impregnated plastic intrauterine device
Barnes'
B. curve
B. zone
baroreceptor
baroreflex response

Barr body
barrel-shaped
b.-s. cervix
b.-s. lesion
barren
barrier
b. contraception
b. contraceptive
INTERCEED absorbable adhesion b.
placental b.
bartholinitis
Bartholin's
B. abscess
B. cyst
B. cystectomy
B. duct
B. gland
B. gland carcinoma
Barton's forceps
Bart's
hemoglobin B.
barymazia
basal
b. artery
b. body temperature
b. cell carcinoma
b. plate
baseline
b. fetal heart rate
b. tonus
b. variability of fetal heart rate
Basis soap
bath
sitz b.
battered
b. fetus syndrome
b. wife syndrome
b. woman
battering cycle
battledore placenta
Baudelocque's
B. diameter
B. operation
B. uterine circle
Baumberger forceps
Bayer Timed-Release-Arthritic Pain Formula
Bayley-Pinneau table
BCDDP
Breast Cancer Detection Demonstration Project
BCG
Bacille bilié de Calmette-Guérin
bacillus Calmette-Guérin
BCG vaccination
BCG vaccine
bead-chain cystourethrography
beading
bean
castor b.
bearing down
bearing-down pain
beat-to-beat
b.-t.-b. variability
b.-t.-b. variation of fetal heart rate
Because
Beckwith-Wiedemann syndrome
beclomethasone
Beclovent
Beconase
bed
arterial vascular b.
pulmonary vascular b.
b. rest
Bednar's aphthae
Beesix
belief
pregnancy b.
belladonna
Bellergal
Bell's
B. palsy
B. staging criteria
Benadryl
Benahist
Bendectin
Bendopa
bendroflumethiazide
Benemid
benign
b. breast disease
b. cyst
b. cystic ovarian teratoma
b. gynecologic lesion
b. lesion
b. mass
b. mesothelioma of genital tract
b. nevus
b. ovarian neoplasm
b. ovarian tumor
b. *Papillomavirus* infection
Benoject

benzathine benzylpenicillin
Benzedrine
benzodiazepine
benzoin
benzthiazide
benztropine mesylate
Benzylpenicillin
Berger's renal disease
beta
  b. error
  b. interferon
  b. ray
  transforming growth factor b. (TGFβ)
beta-adrenergic, β-adrenergic agonist, β-adrenergic
  b.-a. agent
  b.-a. agonist
  b.-a. drug
  b.-a. receptor
beta$_2$-adrenergic agent
beta-blocker
beta carotene
Betadine
beta-endorphin, β-endorphin
beta-glucuronidase
beta-hemolytic streptococci
beta-lactam
  b.-l. antibiotic
  b.-l. antimicrobial
beta-lactamase-resistant antistaphylococcal antibiotic
Betalin S
beta-lipotrophin
Betaloc
betamethasone
  b. valerate
Betapen-VK
beta-subunit
  human chorionic gonadotropin b.-s. (β-HCG)
betatron
Betaxin
bethanechol
Bethesda system
Betke-Kleihauer test
Betke stain
Betnelan
Bewon
Bexophene
Biamine
bias
  detection b.
bicarbonate
  b. administration
  sodium b.
bicarbonate-carbonic acid system
Bicillin
Bicillin L.-A.
Bicitra
bicornate uterus
bidiscoidal placenta
bifid uterus
biforate uterus
bigeminal pregnancy
bigeminy
  atrial b.
biischial diameter
bilateral
  b. ectopic pregnancy
  b. myocutaneous graft
  b. ovarian neoplasm
  b. salpingo-oophorectomy (BSO)
  b. simultaneous pregnancies
  b. simultaneous tubal pregnancies
  b. uropathy
bile acid
bilirubin
Billings method
Billroth tumor forceps
Bill's maneuver
Bill traction handle forceps
Bilopaque
Biloptin
bimanual
  b. pelvic examination
  b. version
binder
  obstetrical b.
binding
  breast b.
  fragment antigen b.
  protein b.
  b. protein
  b. site
bioactive
  b. follicle-stimulating hormone
  b. luteinizing hormone
bioassay
biochemical study
biochemistry
biofeedback therapy

biologic
- b. assay
- b. response modifier (BRM)

Biomydrin
biophysical profile
biopsy
- aspiration b.
- cervical cone b.
- chorionic villus b.
- cone b.
- b. dating
- endometrial b.
- excision b.
- fine-needle aspiration b.
- Kevorkian punch b.
- Keyes punch b.
- kidney b.
- needle b.
- out-of-phase endometrial b.
- outpatient b.
- punch b.
- renal b.
- vulvar b.

biosynthesis
- prostaglandin b.
- steroid b.

biosynthetic defect
Biotirmone
biparietal diameter (BPD)
bipartite
- b. uterus

biperiden
biphenyl
- polychlorinated b.

bipolar
- b. taxis
- b. version

Bird's vacuum extractor
Birnberg bow
birth
- b. amputation
- b. asphyxia
- b. canal
- b. canal laceration
- b. care center
- b. certificate
- b. control
- b. control pill
- b. defect
- b. fracture
- home b.
- hospital b.
- b. injury
- b. interval control
- multiple b.
- b. place
- premature b.
- preterm b.
- b. rate
- b. trauma
- twin b.
- b. weight

bisacodyl
biscoumacetate
- ethyl b.

bishydroxycoumarin
bitartrate
- dihydrocodeine b.

bitemporal diameter
bivalent chromosome
bivalve speculum
black
- b. jaundice
- b. line

bladder
- b. catheter
- b. dysfunction
- b. function
- b. laceration
- b. muscle stress test
- b. neck
- b. neck elevation test
- b. neck mobility
- b. neck suspension
- b. retractor
- b. retraining
- b. tumor
- urinary b.

blade
- Balfour bladder b.

blanching
- laser b.

blastocyst
blastomere
blastomycosis
blastula
bleeder in tumor mass
bleeding
- abnormal uterine b.
- anovulatory b.
- antepartum b.
- breakthrough b.
- dysfunctional uterine b. (DUB)
- estrogen breakthrough b.

estrogen-progesterone withdrawal b.
estrogen withdrawal b.
intermenstrual b.
packing for b.
painless vaginal b.
pelvic b.
postmenarchal b.
postmenopausal b.
preadolescent vaginal b.
progesterone breakthrough b.
progesterone withdrawal b.
b. site
b. site ligation
third trimester b.
b. time
uterine b.
vaginal b.
withdrawal b.

blennorrhagia

blennorrhagic

blennorrhea

blennorrheal

Blenoxane

bleomycin
cisplatin, vinblastine, and b.

Bleph-10

blighted ovum

Blocadren

block
atrioventricular b.
complete heart b.
congenital heart b.
extradural b.
heart b.
nerve b.
paracervical b.
pudendal b.
saddle b.
subarachnoid b.

blockade
spinal b.

blockage
proximal tubal b.

blocker
adrenergic b.
alpha-adrenergic b.
calcium channel b.
cyproheptadine receptor b.
ganglionic b.

blocking factor

blood
b. analysis
autologous b.
b. chimerism
b. component
cord b.
b. count
fetal b.
b. flow
b. gas
b. glucose
b. group
intervillous b.
b. loss
maternal b.
maternal peripheral b.
b. mole
oxygenated fetal b.
b. patch
b. pigment staining
b. pressure
b. product
b. spots
b. study
b. sugar
b. sugar monitoring
b. transfusion
b. urea nitrogen (BUN)
b. vessel formation
b. volume
whole b.

blood-type test

bloody show

Bloom's syndrome

blot
Southern b.
Western b.

Blue
Azovan B.
Urolene B.

blue
b. asphyxia
b. baby
b. dome cyst
methylene b.
toluidine b.

blueberry muffin baby

blues
postpartum b.

blunt
b. duct adenosis
b. trauma

B-mode ultrasound

body
Barr b.

body *(continued)*
  Call-Exner b.
  dense b.
  Döhle b.
  Donovan b.
  b. fluid
  foreign b.
  b. mass index
  b. mass index nomogram
  perineal b.
  polar b.
  psammoma b.
  Schiller-Duvall b.
  b. stalk
  b. surface area calculation
  b. weight
Bohr effect
Bonamine
bone
  b. accretion
  b. density
  b. estrogen receptor
  b. formation
  innominate b.
  b. loss
  b. marrow
  b. marrow failure
  b. marrow toxicity
  b. marrow transplantation
  b. mass
  b. mineral content
  b. mineral density
  b. pain
  b. resorption
  b. tumor
  b. turnover
  weight-bearing b.
Bonine
Bonney's test
Bontril
bony metastasis
booster
  tetanus toxoid b.
borderline
  b. epithelial ovarian carcinoma
  b. epithelial ovarian neoplasm
  b. epithelial ovarian tumor
  b. malignant epithelial neoplasm
  b. ovarian serous tumor
  b. ovarian tumor
boric acid
Borrelia burgdorferi
botryoid
  b. pseudosarcoma
  b. sarcoma
Bouin's solution
bound
  b. estradiol
  b. testosterone
bow
  Birnberg b.
bowel
  b. function
  b. habits
  b. obstruction
  b. preparation
  small b.
  b. sounds
bowenoid
  b. atypia
  b. papulosis
Bozeman
  B. dressing forceps
Bozeman-Fritsch catheter
Bozeman's operation
BPD
  biparietal diameter
brachial
  b. birth palsy
  b. plexus
  b. plexus injury
Bracht maneuver
brachypellic, brachypelvic
brachytherapy
bradycardia
  fetal b.
  sinus b.
bradykinin
bradymenorrhea
bradytocia
Bragg peak
brain
  b. damage
  b. damage indicator
  b. death
  b. disorder
  fetal b.
  b. peptide
  b. sparing
brain-death syndrome
2-Br-alpha-ergocryptine mesylate
Brandt-Andrews maneuver
Braun episiotomy scissors

Braune's canal
Braun-Schroeder single-tooth tenaculum
brawny arm
Braxton-Hicks
B.-H. contraction
B.-H. sign
B.-H. version
breach of duty
breakdown
endometrial b.
wound b.
breakthrough bleeding
breast
accessory b.
adenoma of b.
adolescent b.
augmented b.
b. binding
b. biopsy tissue
caked b.
b. cancer
b. cancer prevalence
b. carcinoma
b. care
b. change
childhood b.
compression of b.'s
b. cyst
cystic disease of b.
b. discomfort
b. disease
b. embryology
engorged b.
b. engorgement
fascia of b.
b. feeding
irritable b.
lactating b.
b. milk
b. milk jaundice
nonlactating b.
b. pain
prepubertal development of b.
b. pump
b. self-examination (BSE)
Breast Cancer Detection Demonstration Project (BCDDP)
breathing
fetal b.
breech
b. delivery
b. extraction
b. head
b. presentation
Brenner tumor
Breonesin
Brethaire
Brethine
bretylium tosylate
Bretylol
Breus mole
Brevibloc
Brevicon
Bricanyl
Bricker procedure
brittle diabetes
BRM
biologic response modifier
broad
b. ligament
b. ligament hematoma
b. ligament pregnancy
bromide
ammonium b.
calcium b.
distigmine b.
mepenzolate b.
methantheline b.
Peacock's b.
potassium b.
sodium b.
strontium b.
Triple b.
bromocriptine
injectable b.
b. resistance
b. therapy
bromocriptine-resistant prolactinoma
bromodiphenhydramine
bromopheniramine maleate
bromsulfophthalein (BSP)
bronchial asthma
bronchiectasis
bronchitis
bronchopulmonary dysplasia
bronchoscopy
Bronitin Mist
Bronkaid
Bronkephrine
Bronkodyl
Bronkometer
Bronkosol
brow presentation
Brunschwig's operation

brush
endocervical sampling b.
B-scanner
real-time B.-s.
static B.-s.
BSE
breast self-examination
BSO
bilateral salpingo-oophorectomy
BSP
bromsulfophthalein
bubble stability test
bubo
bullet b.
chancroidal b.
climatic b.
primary b.
tropical b.
venereal b.
virulent b.
bubonic
Bucladin-S softabs
buclizine
bud
syncytial b.
taste b.
Buddha stance
Buffaprin
buffered aspirin
Bufferin
Buffinol
buffy coat component
bulb
sinovaginal b.
vestibular b.
bulbitis
bulbocavernosus
b. fat flap
b. muscle
bulbourethral gland
bulimia
b. nervosa
bulky cervical carcinoma
bullet bubo
BUN
blood urea nitrogen
bupivacaine
buprenorphine hydrochloride
Burch
B. colposuspension
B. procedure
burden
tumor b.
burning vulvar syndrome
Burow's solution
bursa-dependent system
bursa of Fabricius
buserelin
busulfan, busulphan
Butalan
butalbital
Butalgen
Butanefrine
butaperazine
Butazolidin
Butazone
butoconazole
butorphanol
butoxide pyrethrins and piperonyl
butriptyline hydrochloride
butyrophenone
bypass
cardiopulmonary b.
gastric b.
jejunoileal b.
b. surgery

C

CA-125
  cancer antigen-125
CA-125 assay
cachectin
CAF
  cyclophosphamide, doxorubicin, and 5-fluorouracil
café au lait spot
caffeine
caked breast
Calan
calcifediol
Calciferol
calcification
  arterial c.
  coarse c.
  dystrophic c.
  granulomatous c.
  malignant c.
  popcorn-like c.
  skin c.
  sutural c.
  vascular c.
Calcimar
Calciparine
calcitonin
calcitriol
calcitropic hormone
calcium
  c. absorption
  c. agonist
  c. antagonist
  c. bromide
  c. channel blocker
  c. cyclamate
  docusate c.
  c. heparin
  c. ion
  microcysts of milk of c.
  c. pantothenate
  c. supplement
  c. supplementation
calculation
  body surface area c.
calculus, gen. and pl. **calculi**
  mammary c.
  renal calculi
  urinary c.
  uterine c.
Calderol
Caldwell-Moloy classification
calf
  c. pain
  c. vein thrombosis
californium
californium-252 (^{252}Cf)
calipers
Calkins' sign
Call-Exner body
Calmette-Guérin
  bacillus C.-G. (BCG)
calmodulin
calorie
Calymmatobacterium granulomatis
cAMP
  cyclic adenosine monophosphate
camphor
camphorated oil
camsylate
  trimethaphan c.
canal
  Alcock's c.
  anal c.
  birth c.
  Braune's c.
  cervical c.
  endocervical c.
  inguinal c.
  neurenteric c.
  Nuck's c.
  parturient c.
  uterovaginal c.
canalicular period
canaliculus
cancer
  breast c.
  cervical c.
  cervical stump c.
  c. chemotherapy
  colorectal c.
  endometrial c.
  epithelial c.
  gynecologic c.
  intraepithelial endometrial c.
  invasive c.
  invasive cervical c.
  lung c.
  microinvasive cervical c.
  occult c.
  ovarian c.

cancer *(continued)*
rectal c.
c. and steroid hormone (CASH)
testicular c.
c. therapy
thyroid c.
vaginal c.
cancer antigen-125 (CA-125)
Cancer Committee of College of American Pathologists
Candida
C. albicans
C. glabrata
C. tropicalis
C. vaginitis
candidiasis
vaginal c.
vulvovaginal c.
Canesten
cannabis
cannula
Karmen c.
Cantil
Cantor tube
CAP
cyclophosphamide, doxorubicin, cisplatin
cap
cervical c.
Dutch c.
capacitation
sperm c.
capacity
corticosteroid-binding globulin-binding c. (CBG-BC)
fetal blood oxygen-carrying c.
functional residual c.
lung c.
maximum breathing c.
oxygen-diffusing c.
plasma iron-binding c.
pulmonary diffusing c.
urinary concentrating c.
vital c.
capillary blood sampling
Capoten
capped uterus
caproate
hydroxyprogesterone c.
17-hydroxyprogesterone c.
17α-hydroxyprogesterone c.
capsularis
capsule
Heyman's c.'s
captopril
capture
ovum c.
caput, gen. **capitis**, pl. **capita**
c. succedaneum
carbachol
carbamazepine
Carbamide
carbarsone
carbazole
carbenicillin
carbimazole
carbinoxamine maleate
carbohydrate
c. intolerance
c. metabolism
c. tolerance
Carbolith
carbon
c. dioxide (CO_2)
c. dioxide gas
c. dioxide laser
c. dioxide tension
c. monoxide poisoning
carbonic acid
carboplatin
carboxamide
dimethyl-triazeno-imidazole c. (DTIC)
carcinoembryonic
c. antigen (CEA)
c. antigen-125 (CEA-125)
carcinogen
chemical c.
carcinoid
carcinoma, pl. **carcinomas, carcinomata**
adenoid cystic c.
adenosquamous c.
advanced c.
anaplastic c.
Bartholin's gland c.
basal cell c.
borderline epithelial ovarian c.
breast c.
bulky cervical c.
cecal c.

cervical c.
clear cell endometrial c.
colloid c.
colon c.
contralateral synchronous c.
ductal c.
early vulvar c.
embryonal c.
endometrial c.
endometrioid c.
epithelial ovarian c.
fallopian tube c.
focal lobular c.
glassy cell c.
gynecological c.
hepatocellular c.
infiltrating c.
infiltrating small cell lobular c.
inflammatory c.
intracystic papillary c.
intraductal c.
intraductal papillary c.
invasive c.
juvenile c.
lobular c.
lung c.
medullary c.
mesometanephric c.
mesonephric c.
metaplastic c.
metastatic c.
microinvasive c.
mucinous c.
multicentric c.
ovarian c.
ovarian small cell c.
papillary c.
papillary endometrial c.
papillary serous cervical c.
preclinical c.
recurrent c.
renal cell c.
scirrhous c.
secretory c.
signet ring cell c.
squamous cell c.
tubular c.
uterine papillary serous c.
vaginal c.
verrucous c.
vulvar c.
vulvovaginal c.
well-circumscribed c.
Wolfe classification of breast c.
wolffian duct c.

carcinoma in situ

carcinosarcoma

uterine c.

cardiac

c. anomaly
c. arrest
c. arrhythmia
c. care
c. disease
c. dysrhythmia
c. failure
c. function
c. glycoside
c. massage
c. output

Cardilate

cardinal

c. ligament
c. movements
c. points

cardiogenic shock

cardiomyopathy

peripartum c.
postpartum c.

cardiopulmonary

c. bypass
c. collapse
c. disorder
c. resuscitation

Cardioquin

cardiorespiratory function

cardiotachometer

cardiotocography

intrapartum c.

cardiovascular

c. adverse effect
c. complication
c. disease
c. effect
c. system

care

ambulatory c.
antepartum c.
breast c.
cardiac c.
follow-up c.
health c.
obstetrical c.
postoperative c.

care *(continued)*
postpartum c.
preconception c.
prenatal c.
prepregnancy c.
caries
dental c.
Carmol
carneous
c. degeneration
c. mole
carnitine
carotid artery
carotin
carpal tunnel syndrome
carphenazine maleate
carrier
fragile X c.
heterozygous c.
Miya hook ligature c.
c. protein
translocation c.
caruncle
amnionic c.
myrtiform c.
urethral c.
caruncula, pl. **carunculae**
c. hymenalis, pl. carunculae hymenales
c. myrtiformis, pl. carunculae myrtiformes
Carus'
C. circle
C. curve
casanthranol
cascara sagrada
case
index c.
c. report
CASH
cancer and steroid hormone
CASH study
cast
decidual c.
castor bean
castrate
castration
CAT
computed axial tomography
catagen phase
catamenia
catamenial
catamenogenic
Catapres
cat-cry syndrome
catecholamine
endogenous c.
c. reduction
catechol estrogen
catgut suture
cathartic
saline c.
catheter
bladder c.
Bozeman-Fritsch c.
central venous c.
Davis bladder c.
double-balloon c.
Drew-Smythe c.
female c.
femoral arterial c.
Foley c.
percutaneous nephrostomy c.
peritoneal c.
suction c.
Swan-Ganz c.
Word bladder c.
catheterization
femoral artery c.
pulmonary artery c.
catheter-within-a-catheter
caudal
c. analgesia
c. anesthesia
c. regression syndrome
caul
cautery
c. conization
laparoscopic c.
ovarian c.
cava
inferior vena c.
superior vena c.
vena c.
cavernous plexus
cavity
amniotic c.
oral c.
C band
CBG
corticosteroid-binding globulin
CBG-BC
corticosteroid-binding globulin-binding capacity
CDC
Centers for Disease Control

CD_4 cell
CD_8 cell
CDE blood group system
cDNA
complementary DNA
CEA
carcinoembryonic antigen
CEA-125
carcinoembryonic antigen-125
cecal carcinoma
Ceclor
Cecon
Cedilanid
Cedilanid-D
Cedocard-SR
cefaclor
cefadroxil
Cefadyl
cefamandole
cefazolin
Cefizox
Cefobid
cefonicid
cefoperazone
ceforanide
cefotaxime
cefotetan
cefoxitin sodium
ceftazimide
ceftizoxime
ceftriaxone
cefuroxime
celiohysterectomy
celiohysterotomy
celiomyomectomy
celiomyomotomy
celiosalpingectomy
celiosalpingotomy
celiotomy
vaginal c.
cell
antigen-sensitive c.
B c.
c. block analysis
c. carcinoma of cervix
CD_4 c.
CD_8 c.
committed c.
c. culture
c. cycle
c. cycling in chemotherapy
cytotoxic c.
decidual c.
double c. (D cell)
effector c.
endothelial c.
fetal c.
frozen red c.
c. generation time
germ c.
granulosa c.
granulosa lutein c.
c. growth inhibitor
helper T c.
hobnail c.'s
Hofbauer c.
immunocompetent c.
interstitial c.
K c.
c. kill
killer c.
c. kinetics
koilocytotic c.
Langerhans' c.'s
Langhans' c.'s
Leydig's c.'s
lipid c.
lutein c.
lymphoid c.
lymphokine-activated killer c. (LAK)
memory c.
mutant c.
myoepithelial c.
natural killer c.'s (NK cells)
osteoblast-like c.
packed c.'s
pituitary c.
placental giant c.
pregnancy c.
primordial germ c.
red blood c.
Sertoli-Leydig c.
Sertoli's c.
squamous c.
steroid c.
suppressor c.
suppressor T c.
c. surface antigen
T c.
target c.
theca c.
thecal/interstitial c.
theca lutein c.
trophoblastic c.

cell *(continued)*
  tuboendometrial c.
  white blood c.
cell-mediated immunity (CMI)
cellular
  c. cytotoxic mechanism
  c. division
  c. immunity
  c. migration
cellulitic phlegmasia
cellulitis
  pelvic c.
Celontin
Cemill
Cenafed
Cena-K
center
  birth care c.
  epiphyseal ossification c.
  lower limb ossification c.
Centers for Disease Control (CDC)
central
  c. axis depth dose
  c. defect
  c. nervous system (CNS)
  c. nervous system abnormality
  c. nervous system differentiation
  c. nervous system tumor
  c. neurologic adverse effect
  c. placenta previa
  c. venous catheter
  c. venous pressure (CVP)
centromere
cephalexin
cephalhematoma
cephalic
  c. forceps
  c. pole
  c. presentation
  c. replacement
  c. version
cephalohematoma
cephalometry
  ultrasonic c.
cephalopelvic
  c. disproportion
cephalopelvimetry
cephalosporin
cephalothin
cephalotome
cephalotomy
cephalotribe
cephapirin
cephradine
Cephulac
Ceporex
cerclage
  cervical c.
  Mann isthmic c.
  McDonald cervical c.
  Shirodkar cervical c.
  transabdominal cervicoisthmic c.
cerebellar degeneration
cerebral
  c. angioma
  c. blood flow
  c. dysfunction
  c. edema
  c. embolism
  c. infarction
  c. palsy
  c. palsy antecedent
  c. palsy prevention
  c. palsy risk
  c. thrombosis
  c. venous thrombosis
cerebral-placental ratio
cerebrospinal fluid
cerebrovascular
  c. accident (CVA)
  c. disease
Cerespan
certificate
  birth c.
Cerubidine
ceruloplasmin
cervical
  c. abnormality
  c. amputation
  c. anomaly
  c. artery
  c. canal
  c. cancer
  c. cap
  c. carcinoma
  c. carcinoma screening
  c. carcinoma stimulation
  c. cerclage
  c. clear cell adenocarcinoma
  c. cone biopsy
  c. conization
  c. culture

c. cytology
c. dilation
c. dysplasia
c. ectopic pregnancy
c. ectropion
c. effacement
c. epithelial neoplasia
c. epithelium
c. erosion
c. eversion
c. factor
c. GIFT
c. Gram stain
c. incision
c. incompetence (CI)
c. infection
c. insemination
c. intraepithelial neoplasia (CIN)
c. laceration
c. leiomyoma
c. leiomyosarcoma
c. lesion
c. mucorrhea
c. mucus
c. myoma
c. neoplasia
c. os
c. *Papillomavirus*
c. Pap smear
c. polyp
c. pregnancy
c. priming
c. prolapse
c. ripening
c. sarcoma
c. stenosis
c. stroma
c. stump cancer
c. stump tumor
c. transformation zone
c. zone

cervicectomy

cervicitis
gonorrheal c.
mucopurulent c.

cervicography

cervicoplasty

cervicotomy

cervicovaginal
c. infection
c. ridge

cervix
atretic c.
barrel-shaped c.
cell carcinoma of c.
cone biopsy of c.
conization of c.
dilation of c.
incompetent c.
international classification of cancer of c.
malignant tumor of c.
multiple c.

cesarean
c. delivery
c. hysterectomy
c. operation
repeat c.
c. section (C-section)
c. section hemorrhage
c. section rate
c. section scar

cesium

cesium-137 (^{137}Cs)

cesium-137 level

cessation

Cetamide

Cetane

Cevalin

Cevi-Bid

Ce-Vi-Sol

Cevita

^{252}Cf
californium-252

c-fms proto-oncogene

CG
chorionic gonadotropin

Chadwick's sign

challenge
intravenous glucose c.
progestational c.

Chamberlen forceps

chancroid

chancroidal bubo

change
atrophic c.
breast c.
concomitant c.
fibrocystic c.
fibrocystic breast c.
focal c.
glomerular c.
hematological c.

change *(continued)*
- hormone-stimulated endometrial c.
- immunohistochemical c.
- immunologic c.
- libidinal c.
- c. of life
- ovarian cycle c.
- postbiopsy c.
- posttherapy c.
- retinal c.
- sensorineural c.
- visual c.

channel
- surface epithelium vascular c.
- vascular c.

characteristic
- epidemiological c.
- morphological c.
- secondary sex c.

characterization
- immunohistochemical stromal leukocyte c.

chart
- Babson c.
- Ballard c.
- basal body temperature c.
- pedigree c.
- Walker's c.

Chassar moir sling procedure

chemical
- c. carcinogen
- c. pneumonitis
- c. pregnancy

chemiluminescent immunoassay (CIA)

chemoimmunotherapy

chemoprophylaxis

chemoreceptor

chemotactic factor

chemotherapeutic
- c. agent
- c. treatment

chemotherapy
- adjuvant c.
- alkylating c.
- cancer c.
- cell cycling in c.
- combination c.
- high-dose c.
- intraperitoneal c.
- intraperitoneal cisplatin c.
- Karnofsky performance status of c.
- metabolism in intraperitoneal c.
- c. phase trial
- postoperative c.
- prophylactic c.

chest
- c. examination
- c. radiography

Chiari-Frommel syndrome

chiasma, pl. **chiasmata**
- c. formation

chickenpox
- c. pneumonia

child
- c. abuse
- unborn c.

childbearing
- c. age

childbed fever

childbirth
- natural c.
- physiologic c.

childhood
- c. breast
- c. genital trauma

chimera

chimerism
- blood c.

Chlamydia
- *C. psittaci*
- *C. trachomatis*

chlamydial
- c. conjunctivitis
- c. infection
- c. vaginitis

Chlo-Amine

chloasma

Chlor-100

chloral hydrate

chlorambucil

chloramphenicol

chlorcyclizine hydrochloride

chlordiazepoxide
- c. hydrochloride

chloride
- ammonium c.
- oxybutynin c.
- potassium c.
- pralidoxime c.
- sodium c.

chlormethiazole

Chlor-Niramine
Chlorohist-LA
chloroprocaine hydrochloride
chloroquine
chlorothiazide
chlorotrianisene
chlorpheniramine
Chlor-Pro
Chlorpromanyl
chlorpromazine
chlorpropamide
chlorprothixene
Chlortab
chlortetracycline
chlorthalidone
Chlor-Trimeton
Chlor-Tripolon
chlorzoxazone
choanal atresia
chocolate cyst
cholangiopancreatography
    endoscopic retrograde c.
Cholebrine
cholecalciferol
cholecystectomy
cholecystitis
cholecystokinin
Choledyl
cholelithiasis
cholera vaccine
cholestasis
    maternal c.
cholestatic
    c. hepatosis of pregnancy
    c. jaundice
cholesterol
cholesterolemia
    familial c.
cholesterol ester storage disease
cholestyramine
choline
    c. salicylate
    c. theophyllinate
cholinergic
    c. agonist
    c. drug
cholinesterase
    c. inhibitor
Choloxin
chondroectodermal dysplasia
chondrosarcoma
    uterine c.
chorda, pl. **chordae**
    c. umbilicalis
chorea
    c. gravidarum
chorioadenoma
    c. destruens
chorioallantoic
    c. placenta
    c. vessel
chorioamnionic
    c. infection
    c. placenta
chorioamnionitis
    Gardnerella vaginalis c.
chorioamniotic infection
chorioangioma
chorioangiomatosis
chorioangiosis
choriocarcinoma
choriogonadotropin
chorion
    c. frondosum
    c. laeve
chorionic
    c. adrenocorticotropin
    c. cyst
    c. gonadotrophic hormone
    c. gonadotrophin
    c. gonadotropic hormone
    c. gonadotropin (CG)
    c. growth hormone
    c. thyrotropin
    c. vascularization
    c. vesicle
    c. villi
    c. villus biopsy
    c. villus sampling (CVS)
chorioretinitis
Christmas disease
chromatid
    sister c.
chromatin
    sex c.
chromatography
    thin-layer c.
chromic
    c. gut pelviscopic loop ligature
    c. phosphate
chromosomal
    c. abnormality

chromosomal *(continued)*
c. analysis
c. anomaly
c. banding
c. deletion
c. pattern
c. sex
c. structural abnormality
c. translocation
chromosome
c. 21
c. abnormality
bivalent c.
fragile X c.
long arm of c.
c. mosaicism
Philadelphia c.
sex c.
c. triploidy
X c.
XX c.
Y c.
chronic
c. atrophic vulvitis
c. cystic mastitis
c. fetal hypoxia
c. hepatitis
c. hypertension
c. hypertrophic vulvitis
c. interstitial salpingitis
c. pelvic pain
c. scrotal hypothermia
c. vascular disease
Chronulac
chylomicron
CI
cervical incompetence
CIA
chemiluminescent immunoassay
ciclopirox
CI Direct Blue #53
Cidomycin
CI Food Blue #1
cigarette smoking
ciliated metaplasia
cilium, pl. **cilia**
cimetidine
CIN
cervical intraepithelial neoplasia
cinnarizine
Cinobac
cinoxacin
Cin-Quin
ciprofloxacin
circadian
c. cycle
c. rhythm
circle
Baudelocque's uterine c.
Carus' c.
circulating
c. luteinizing hormone
c. platelet antibody
circulation
fetal c.
fetoplacental c.
hypophyseal portal c.
hypothalamic-hypophyseal portal c.
persistent fetal c.
c. time
umbilical c.
circumcise
circumcision
circumference
abdominal c.
fetal abdominal c.
midarm c.
circumflex artery
circumscribed mass
cirrhonosus
cirrhosis
hypertrophic c.
c. of liver
cisplatin
intraperitoneal c.
c. nephrotoxicity
c. neutralization
cissa
citrate
clomiphene c.
fentanyl c.
magnesium c.
potassium c.
sufentanil c.
tamoxifen c.
citrovorum
c. factor
citrullinemia
citta, cittosis
Claforan
claim
malpractice c.
non-obstetrical c.
obstetrical c.

clamp
- Allis c.
- Babcock c.
- Backhaus c.
- Ballentine c.
- DeBakey c.
- Heaney c.
- Kelly c.
- Kocher c.
- mogen c.
- pedicle c.
- Pennington c.
- thoracic c.
- Willett's c.

Clark classification of vulvar melanoma

class
- c. I receptor
- c. II receptor
- c. A diabetes

classical
- c. cesarean section
- c. transverse incision

classification
- American Society of Anesthesiologists c.
- Astler-Coller modification of Dukes' c.
- Caldwell-Moloy c.
- Dripps–American Society of Anesthesiologists c.
- Dukes c.
- Federation of Gynecology and Obstetrics c.
- International Federation of Gynecology and Obstetrics c.
- microinvasive carcinoma c.
- tumor nodal metastasis c. (TNM classification)
- Wolfe c. of breast cancer

clathrin

clavulanic acid

clear
- c. cell adenocarcinoma
- c. cell endometrial carcinoma

clearance
- creatinine c.
- immune c.
- urate c.
- urea c.

cleavage
- embryonic c.

cleft
- c. lip
- c. palate

cleidotomy

clemastine

Cleocin

clidinium

clidoic

climacteric
- grand c.
- c. psychosis
- c. syndrome

climacterium

climatic bubo

clindamycin

clinical
- c. finding
- c. prognosis
- c. staging

clinicopathological analysis

Clinoril

clip
- c. technique
- towel c.

Clistin

clitoridectomy

clitoriditis

clitoris
- c. enlargement

clitorism

clitoritis

clitoromegaly

cloaca

clofibrate

Clomid

clomiphene
- c. citrate
- c. fetal malformation

clomiphene-resistant polycystic ovary syndrome

clomipramine

clomocycline

clonal selection theory

clonazepam

clone
- molecular c.

clonidine

cloning
- gene c.

Clopra

Cloquet's node

clorazepate
closed chest massage
closing volume
Clostridium
  C. perfringens
closure
  incision c.
  premature airway c.
  premature ductus arteriosis c.
  Smead-Jones c.
clot
  retroplacental c.
clothing
clotrimazole
cloxacillin
Cloxapen
clubfoot
clue cell
cluster
CMF
  cyclophosphamide, methotrexate, 5-fluorouracil
CMF(P)
  cyclophosphamide, methotrexate, 5-fluorouracil, and prednisone
CMFVP
  cyclophosphamide, methotrexate, 5-fluorouracil, vincristine, and prednisone
CMI
  cell-mediated immunity
c-*myc* gene
CNS
  central nervous system
CNS development
CO_2
  carbon dioxide
^{60}Co
  cobalt-60
coagulation
  cold c.
  c. defect
  c. disorder
  disseminated intravascular c. (DIC)
  c. factor
  c. profile
  c. test
coagulator
  argon beam c.
  cold c.
coagulopathy
  consumption c.
  maternal c.
coarctation of aorta
coarse calcification
cobalt
  c. megavoltage machine
cobalt-60 (^{60}Co)
Cobantril
cocaine
  c. addiction
  perinatal c.
coccidiomycosis
coccus, pl. **cocci**
  Gram-positive cocci
coccygodynia
coccyx
cocktail
  pediatric c.
code
  genetic c.
codeine
codon
coefficient of variation (CV)
coelom
coelomic
  c. epithelium
  c. metaplasia
coexistent fetus
coffee
Coffey suspension
Cogentin
coil
  metal c.
coiled artery
coital
  c. factor
coition
coitus
  c. interruptus
Colace
Colax
colchicine
cold
  c. coagulation
  c. coagulator
  common c.
  c. conization
  c. knife conization
coleitis
coleocele
coleotomy

colic
c. artery
meconial c.
menstrual c.
ovarian c.
tubal c.
uterine c.
colistimethate sodium
colistin
colitis
pseudomembranous c.
ulcerative c.
collagen
c. disease
microfibrillar c.
c.-vascular disease
collapse
cardiopulmonary c.
collapsed subpectoral implant
collateral
venous c.
Colles' fracture
collimator
colloid
c. carcinoma
c. osmotic pressure (COP)
radioactive c.
colon
c. carcinoma
sigmoid c.
colonic obstruction
colonoscopy
colony-stimulating factor
colorectal
c. anastomosis
c. cancer
c. cancer endoscopy
c. tumor
colostomy
diverting c.
fecal diversion c.
temporary diverting c.
colostration
colostric
colostrorrhea
colostrous
colostrum
colovaginal fistula
colpatresia
colpectasis, colpectasia
colpectomy
colpitis
c. mycotica
colpocele
colpocleisis
colpocystitis
colpocystocele
colpocystoplasty
colpocystotomy
colpocystoureterotomy
colpodynia
colpohyperplasia
c. cystica, c. emphysematosa
colpohysterectomy
colpohysteropexy
colpohysterotomy
colpomicroscope
colpomicroscopy
colpomycosis
colpomyomectomy
colpopathy
colpoperineoplasty
colpoperineorrhaphy
colpopexy
colpoplasty
colpopoiesis
colpoptosis, colpoptosia
colporectopexy
colporrhagia
colporrhaphy
colporrhexis
colposcope
colposcopic
c. diagnosis
c. screening
c. view
colposcopy
endocervical canal c.
estrogen-assisted c.
colpospasm
colpostat
colpostenosis
colpostenotomy
colposuspension
Burch c.
colpotomy
c. incision
colpoureterotomy
colpourethrocystopexy
retropubic c.
colpoxerosis
columnar
c. epithelium
c. epithelium papilla
Coly-Mycin
Coly-Mycin M

Coly-Mycin S
coma
combination
c. chemotherapy
estrogen-progestogen c.
norgestrel/ethinyl estradiol c.
combination oral contraceptive
combined
c. birth control pill
c. immunodeficiency
c. pregnancy
c. version
comedocarcinoma
comedo and cribriform form
commissure
posterior c.
commissurotomy
mitral c.
committed cell
common cold
communicating uterus
communication
autocrine c.
fetal-maternal c.
paracrine c.
vascular c.
compacta
compatibility
maternal-fetal HLA c.
Compazine
compelled medical treatment
complement
c. fixation
c. value
complementary DNA (cDNA)
complete
c. abortion
c. breech presentation
c. heart block
c. hydatidiform mole
c. precocious puberty
c. remission
complex
AIDS dementia c. (ADC)
AIDS-related c. (ARC)
antigen-antibody c.
tubo-ovarian c.
vitamin B c.
compliance
lung c.
complication
cardiovascular c.
neurologic c.
obstetrical c.
operative site c.
postoperative c.
pregnancy c.
pulmonary c.
respiratory c.
vascular c.
component
blood c.
buffy coat c.
extensive intraductal c. (EIC)
compound
c. nevus of vulva
nitroimidazole c.
c. pregnancy
c. presentation
compressibility
vein c.
compression
c. of breasts
cord c.
c. device
external pneumatic calf c. (EPC)
c. force
head c.
pneumatic c.
spot c.
uterine c.
compressus
fetus c.
Compton effect
computed
c. axial tomography (CAT)
c. tomographic pelvimetry
c. tomography (CT)
concealed hemorrhage
concentrate
factor c.
platelet c.
concentration
fetal steroid c.
inhibin c.
lipoprotein c.
maternal steroid c.
mean hemoglobin c.
mean plasma iron c.
plasma iron c.
serum c.
serum lithium c.
steroid c.

conception
assisted c.
estimated date of c. (EDC)
natural c.
wrongful c.
Conceptrol
conceptus, pl. **concepti**
concomitant change
condition
fetal c.
local ovarian c.
maternal c.
neonatal c.
orthopaedic c.
X-linked dominant c.
X-linked recessive c.
condom
conductance
airway c.
conduction
c. analgesia
c. anesthesia
conduit
ileal c.
intestinal c.
urinary c.
conduplicato corpore
condyloma acuminatum, pl. **condylomata acuminata**
condyloma latum
condylox
cone
c. biopsy
c. biopsy of cervix
transvaginal c.
confidence limits
confinement
estimated/expected date of c. (EDC)
congenital
c. abnormality
c. adrenal hyperplasia
c. adrenal hypoplasia
c. afibrinogenemia
c. amputation
c. anemia
c. anomaly
c. cardiac defect
c. defect
c. ectropion
c. folate malabsorption
c. heart block
c. heart defect
c. heart disease
c. hip dislocation
c. hyperplasia
c. hypofibrinogenemia
c. hypothyroidism
c. injury
c. malformation
c. nephrosis
c. pneumonia
c. postural deformity
c. rubella
c. rubella syndrome
c. spastic paraplegia
c. syphilis
c. toxoplasmosis
congestion
pelvic vein c.
congestive heart failure
conglutination
conization
cautery c.
cervical c.
c. of cervix
cold c.
cold-knife c.
laser cervical c.
loop diathermy cervical c.
conjoined twins
conjugata diagonalis
conjugate
c. axis
diagonal c.
c. diameter of the pelvic inlet
effective c.
external c.
false c.
c. of inlet
internal c.
obstetric c.
obstetric c. of outlet
c. of outlet
true c.
urinary steroid c.
conjugated
c. equine estrogen
c. estrogens
conjunctivitis
chlamydial c.
gonococcal c.
neonatal c.
connection
decidua-macrophage c.

connective
c. tissue
c. tissue disease
c. tissue disorder
consanguinity
consent
informed c.
conservative
c. drug use
c. surgery
consideration
adrenal morphologic c.
constant
association c.
dissociation c.
constipation
constitutional
c. hirsutism
c. precocious puberty
constriction ring
consultation
anesthesiologist c.
consumption
c. coagulopathy
maternal alcohol c.
oxygen c.
contact
mother-child c.
contamination
bacterial c.
content
aspiration of gastric c.'s
bone mineral c.
contiguous gene syndrome
continence
continent
c. ileostomy
c. urinary pouch
continuous
c. epidural analgesia
c. micronized estradiol and progesterone
c. positive airway pressure (CPAP)
c. running monofilament suture
c. subcutaneous insulin infusion
c. subcutaneous insulin injection
continuous/combined treatment
contour
cranial c.
contraception
barrier c.
hormonal c.
injectable c.
long-acting c.
oral c.
postcoital c. (PCC)
postmolar c.
vaginal ring c.
contraceptive
barrier c.
combination oral c.
c. device
c. diaphragm
estrogen-progestin c.
c. failure
injectable c.
intrauterine c. device (IUCD)
c. jelly
long-acting c.
low-dose oral c.
low steroid content combined oral c.
c. method
oral c.
oral steroid c.
ParaGard T380A intrauterine copper c.
progestin oral c.
c. ring
sequential oral c.
c. sponge
steroid c.
c. technique
vaginal c.
contracted pelvis
contraction
Braxton-Hicks c.
myometrial c.
pelvic c.
premature ventricular c. (PVC)
smooth muscle c.
c. stress test
uterine c.
contralateral
c. ovulation
c. synchronous carcinoma
control
birth c.
birth interval c.

glycemic c.
seizure c.
controversy
transfusion c.
conversion
extraglandular c.
convulsion
puerperal c.'s
Cooley's anemia
Coombs' test
cooperativity
theca-granulosa cell c.
Cooper's
C. ligaments
C. suspensory ligaments
COP
colloid osmotic pressure
copper
c. intrauterine device
Copper 7 intrauterine device
Copper T
copulation
cord
c. abnormality
c. blood
c. compression
nephrogenic c.
nuchal c.
c. of Pflüger
sex c.
spinal c.
umbilical c.
vitelline c.
Cordarone
cordate pelvis
cordiform
c. pelvis
c. uterus
cordocentesis
cordotomy
Corgard
Coricidin
corkscrew vessel
cornu, gen. **cornus**, pl. **cornua**
c. uteri
cornual
c. anastomosis
c. pregnancy
coronary
c. artery disease
c. heart disease
c. thrombosis
Coronex
cor pulmonale
corpus, gen. **corporis**, pl. **corpora**
c. albicans cyst
c. fibrosum
c. luteum
c. luteum cyst
c. luteum cyst rupture
c. luteum deficiency syndrome
c. luteum dysfunction
c. luteum function
c. luteum insufficiency
c. luteum size
c. luteum spurium
c. luteum steroidogenesis
c. luteum verum
c. uteri
uterine c.
corpuscle
genital c.
corrective device
Cort enema
cortical
c. granule
c. implantation
c. mass
c. necrosis
c. reaction
c. supremacy stage
corticoid
corticosteroid
fluorinated c.
corticosteroid-binding
c.-b. globulin (CBG)
c.-b. globulin-binding capacity (CBG-BC)
corticosterone
corticotrope
corticotropin-like intermediate lobe peptide
corticotropin-releasing
c.-r. factor
c.-r. hormone (CRH)
c.-r. inhibitor
cortisol
24-hour urinary free c.
c. level
c. response
cortisone
cortol
Cortone
Cortrosyn
Corynebacterium parvum

Cosmegen
cosmetic agent
cosyntropin
co-trimoxazole
Cotte's operation
cotyledon
fetal c.
maternal c.
placental c.
cotyledonary placenta
cough-pressure transmission ratio
Coumadin
coumarin
c. derivative
counseling
divorce c.
drug use c.
genetic c.
count
bacteria c.
blood c.
differential cell c.
erythrocyte c.
leukocyte c.
platelet c.
reticulocyte c.
sperm c.
coupling
receptor c.
court-ordered obstetrical intervention
Couvelaire uterus
cow's milk
Coxsackievirus
C. B
CPAP
continuous positive airway pressure
C_{21} progestin
crab louse
cramp
leg c.
cramping
uterine c.
cranial
c. contour
c. hypertension
craniocaudal view
cranioclasia, cranioclasis
cranioclast
craniopharyngioma
craniotome
craniotomy
C-reactive protein
cream
intravaginal c.
vaginal antibiotic c.
creatinine
c. clearance
Credé's
C. maneuvers
C. methods
cremnocele
crepitus
cretinism
CRH
corticotropin-releasing hormone
crib death
cribriform hymen
cri-du-chat syndrome
Crile
C. forceps
C. hemostat
Crile-Wood needle holder
criminal abortion
crisis
addisonian c.
adrenal c.
hypercalcemic c.
lupus c.
sickle cell c.
crista dividens
criterion, pl. **criteria**
Bell's staging criteria
Spiegelberg's criteria
critical
c. care monitoring
c. weight hypothesis
Crohn's disease
cromolyn sodium
cross-linking
cross-over
cross-reaction
crown-heel length
crowning
crown-rump length
cryocautery
cryoconization
cryoprecipitate
cryopreservation
oocyte c.
cryosurgery
cryotherapy
cryptic hyperandrogenism
cryptococcosis
cryptomenorrhea

cryptorchidism
crystalloid
Reinke's c.'s
crystal violet
Crystapen
Crysticillin AS
Crystodigin
^{137}Cs
cesium-137
C-section
cesarean section
C_{19}-steroid
CT
computed tomography
C-thalassemia
CT pelvimetry
Cu 7
cube type pessary
cul-de-sac
Douglas' c.-d.-s.
rectouterine c.-d.-s.
culdocentesis
nondiagnostic c.
culdoplasty
culdoscope
culdoscopy
culdotomy
Cullen's sign
culture
amniotic fluid cell c.
cell c.
cervical c.
oocyte c.
urine c.
cumulus oophorus
cup
Milex cervical c.
Cuprimine
curage
curet
curettage
dilation and c. (D & C)
endocervical c.
endocervical canal c.
fractional dilation and c.
repeat c.
suction c.
curette, curet
Duncan's c.
Green uterine c.
Heaney c.
Kelly-Gray c.
Kevorkian-Younge c.
Pipelle endometrial suction c.
Randall suction c.
Sims c.
Thomas c.
curettement, curetment
curie
Curtis syndrome
curve
Barnes' c.
Carus' c.
Friedman c.
isodose c.
Liley c.
oxygen dissociation c.
sexual response c.
standard c.
curved hemostat
Cushing's
C. disease
C. syndrome
cutaneous
c. adverse drug effect
c. blood flow
c. lesion
c. melanoma
CV
coefficient of variation
CVA
cerebrovascular accident
CVP
central venous pressure
CVS
chorionic villus sampling
cyanocobalamin
cyanotic heart disease
cybernin
cyclacillin
cyclamate
calcium c.
sodium c.
cyclandelate
cyclase
adenylate c.
cyclazocine
cycle
battering c.
cell c.
circadian c.
duty c.
endometrial c.

cycle *(continued)*
estrogen-progestin artificial c.
fertility c.
genesial c.
intrauterine pressure c.
itch-scratch c.
menstrual c.
menstrual-ovarian c.
ovarian c.
ovulatory c.
postmenarchal c.
reproductive c.
sexual response c.
spontaneous menstrual c.
cycle-nonspecific agent
cycle-specific agent
cyclic
c. adenosine monophosphate (cAMP)
c. proliferative endometrium
cyclic adenosine 3′,5′-monophosphate
cyclic guanosine 3′,5′-monophosphate
cyclizine
c. hydrochloride
c. lactate
cyclopentanoperhydrophenanthrene
cyclopenthiazide
cyclophosphamide
cyclophosphamide, doxorubicin, cisplatin (CAP)
cyclophosphamide, doxorubicin, and 5-fluorouracil (CAF)
cyclophosphamide, methotrexate, 5-fluorouracil (CMF)
cyclophosphamide, methotrexate, 5-fluorouracil, and prednisone (CMF(P))
cyclophosphamide, methotrexate, 5-fluorouracil, vincristine, and prednisone (CMFVP)
cyclopropane
Cyclo-Provera
cycloserine
Cyclospasmol
Cyclosporin A
cyclosporine
cyclothiazide
cycrimine hydrochloride
cyesis
cypionate
estradiol c.
cyproheptadine
c. hydrochloride
c. receptor blocker
cyproterone acetate
cyst
adnexal c.
allantoic c.
apocrine c.
c. aspiration
Bartholin's c.
benign c.
blue dome c.
breast c.
chocolate c.
chorionic c.
corpora lutea c.'s
corpus albicans c.
corpus luteum c.
dermoid c.
dermoid c. of ovary
dysontogenetic c.
echinococcal c.
endometrial c.
epidermal inclusion c.
epithelial c.
fetal ovarian c.
follicular c.
functional ovarian c.
Gartner's c.
inclusion c.
involution c.
lacteal c.
luteal ovarian c.
massive ovarian c.
milk c.
müllerian c.
multilocular c.
multiple c.
nabothian c.
oil c.
oophoritic c.
ovarian c.
paratubal c.
paroophoritic c.
parovarian c.
perimesonephric c.
perimesonephric vaginal c.
posterior fossa c.
rete c. of ovary
sebaceous c.
simple c.

tension c.
theca lutein c.
umbilical c.
urachal c.
vaginal c.
vaginal dysontogenetic c.
vaginal embryonic c.
vaginal inclusion c.
vestibular c.
vitellointestinal c.
vulvar c.
vulvar inclusion c.

cystadenocarcinoma
mucinous c.
ovarian c.
papillary serous c.

cystadenofibroma

cystadenoma
ovarian c.
ovarian proliferative c.
serous c.

cystectomy
Bartholin's c.
ovarian c.
vulvovaginal c.

cystic
c. adnexal mass
c. disease of the breast
c. fibrosis
c. glandular hyperplasia
c. hygroma
c. hyperplasia
c. hyperplasia of the breast
c. hyperplasia photomicrograph
c. kidney
c. mole
c. myoma degeneration

cystinosis

cystinuria

cystitis
bacterial c.
hemorrhagic c.
postoperative c.
postradiation c.
radiation c.

cystocele

cystometrics
office c.

cystometry

cystosarcoma
c. phyllodes

cystoscopy

Cystospaz

cystotomy
suprapubic c.

cystourethrocele

cystourethrography
bead-chain c.
metallic bead chain c.

cystourethropexy
vaginal c.

cystourethroscopy

Cytadren

cytarabine

cytidine
c. diphosphate-choline
c. diphosphate-diacylglycerol
c. monophosphate
c. triphosphate-phosphocholine cytidyltransferase

cytidyltransferase
cytidine triphosphate-phosphocholine c.

cytobrush
spatula c.

cytogenetics

cytogenetic study

cytokine

cytologic screening

cytology
cervical c.
peritoneal c.
vaginal c.

cytomegalic inclusion disease

cytomegalovirus
c. infection

Cytomel

cytophagocytosis

cytophilic antibody

cytopipette

cytoreductive surgery

Cytosar

Cytosar-U

cytosine
c. arabinoside

cytotoxic
c. agent
c. cell
c. effect
c. factor

cytotoxicity

cytotrophoblast
malignant c.

Cytoxan

D

Δ_{450}
D
D cell
double cell
D isoimmunization
dacarbazine
Dacron fiber
dactinomycin
Dagenan
Dalacin C
Dalkon shield
damage
brain d.
hepatocellular d.
obstetrical d.
obturator nerve d.
dAMP
deoxyadenylic acid
danazol
low-dose d.
d. treatment
Dandy-Walker syndrome
Danforth's sign
danger
radiation d.
Danocrine
danthron
D-antigen isoimmunization
dantrolene
Dapa
Daranide
Darbid
Daricon
dark-field
d.-f. examination
d.-f. microscopy
Dartal
Darvocet-N
Darvon
Darvon-N
data
mortality d.
dating
biopsy d.
pregnancy d.
Datril
daunomycin
daunorubicin
DAV
dibromodulcitol with doxorubicin and vincristine
Davis
D. bladder catheter
D. quintuplet
D & C
dilation and curettage
dCMP
deoxycytidylic acid
DDAVP
desmopressin acetate
DDP
cis-diamminedichloroplatinum
D & E
dilation and evacuation
dead fetus syndrome
death
brain d.
crib d.
early embryonic d.
fetal d.
fetal brain d.
infant d.
intrauterine d.
maternal d.
neonatal d.
nonmaternal d.
perinatal d.
single intrauterine d.
Deaver retractor
DeBakey
D. clamp
D. tissue forceps
debendox
Debetrol
debulking
ovarian carcinoma d.
Decadron
decamethonium bromide
decapitate
decapitation
decarboxylase
ornithine d.
pyruvate d.
Decaspray
deceleration
early d.
fetal heart rate d.

deceleration *(continued)*
late d.
variable d.
decidua
d. basalis
d. capsularis
d. compacta
ectopic d.
d. menstrualis
d. parietalis
d. polyposa
tuberous subchorial hematoma of the d.
d. vera
decidual
d. cast
d. cell
d. endometritis
d. prolactin synthesis
d. reaction
decidualized endometrium
decidua-macrophage connection
deciduate placenta
deciduation
deciduitis
deciduoma
Loeb's d.
decline
recurrent premenstrual lithium serum concentration d.
Declomycin
decomposition
decompression
small intestine d.
uterine d.
decongestant
decreased
d. libido
d. mortality
deep
d. circumflex iliac artery
d. vein thrombophlebitis
d. venous thrombosis (DVT)
defect
atrial septal d.
atrioventricular septal d.
biosynthetic d.
birth d.
central d.
coagulation d.
congenital d.
congenital cardiac d.
congenital heart d.
field d.
genitourinary d.
luteal phase d.
neural tube d. (NTD)
ovulatory d.
perineal d.
single-gene d.
ventricular septal d.
defective chorionic vascularization
defeminization
defensive obstetrics
deferoxamine
deficiency
enzyme d.
erythrocyte enzyme d.
factor II d.
factor V d.
factor VII d.
factor IX d.
factor X d.
factor XI d.
factor XIII d.
nonclassic 21-hydroxylase d.
placental sulfatase d.
prostacyclin d.
red cell enzyme d.
skeletal calcium d.
steroid sulfatase d.
thymic-dependent d.
deflexion abnormality
defloration
deformation
deformity
congenital postural d.
hip d.
joint d.
postural d.
degenerating myoma
degeneration
carneous d.
cerebellar d.
cystic myoma d.
hepatolenticular d.
hyaline myoma d.
malignant d.
molar d.
mucoid myoma d.
red d.
sarcomatous myoma d.
degradation

dehiscence
dehydroepiandrosterone (DHEA)
d. sulfate (DHEAS)
d. sulfate loading test
dehydrogenase
20-α-dihydroprogestin d.
17β-estradiol d.
glucose 6-phosphate d.
15-hydroxyprostaglandin d.
3β-hydroxysteroid d.
18-hydroxysteroid d.
lactate d. (LDH)
lactic acid d.
dehydroisoandrosterone
d. sulfate
Deladroxate
Deładumone
Delalutin
delayed
d. first stage
d. hypersensitivity
d. menarche
d. menstruation
d. puberty
DeLee
D. forceps
D. maneuver
D. suctioning
D. universal retractor
Delestrogen
deletion
autosomal d.
chromosomal d.
gene d.
21-hydroxylase gene d.
11p13 chromosome d.
Delfen
delinquency
deliver
delivery
abdominal d.
assisted cephalic d.
breech d.
cesarean d.
Duncan's mechanism of placental d.
forceps d.
high forceps d.
low forceps d.
midforceps d.
d. mode
oxygen d.
postmortem d.
precipitate labor and d.
premature d.
preterm d.
rotational d.
spontaneous cephalic d.
spontaneous preterm d.
twin d.
vacuum extractor d.
vaginal d.
delta
d. agent
d. hepatitis
Deltalin
demecarium
demeclocycline
demedroxyprogesterone acetate (DMPA)
Demerol
4-demethyl-epipodophyllotoxin
Demser
Demulen 1/35
Demulen 1/50
denidation
Denman's spontaneous evolution
dense body
density
arterial linear d.
bone d.
bone mineral d.
fat d.
hip bone d.
dental caries
denticulate hymen
deodorant artifact
deoxyadenylic acid (dAMP)
deoxycorticosterone (DOC)
deoxycytidylic acid (dCMP)
deoxyguanylic acid (dGMP)
deoxyribonucleic acid (DNA)
deoxythymidylic acid (dTMP)
Depakene
Depen
depletion
juvenile spermatogonial d.
Depogen
depo-medroxyprogesterone
Depo-Provera
depression
agitated d.
fetal skull d.
narcotic d.
postpartum d.
respiratory d.

deprivation
antagonist-induced gonadotropin d.
estrogen d.
depth dose
depth-dose distribution
derivation
sexual d.
derivative
acetoxyprogesterone d.
17alpha-acetoxyprogesterone d.
coumarin d.
19-nortestosterone d.
dermatitis, pl. **dermatitides**
atopic d.
papular d. of pregnancy
progesterone d.
seborrheic d.
vulvar contact d.
vulvar seborrheic d.
dermatomyositis
primary idiopathic d.
dermoid
d. cyst
d. cyst of ovary
Deronil
DES
diethylstilbestrol
D. exposure
D. exposure in utero
D. task force
DESAD
National Collaborative Diethylstilbestrol Adenosis Project
descending aorta
descensus
d. uteri
descent
fetal d.
rotation and d.
desensitization
pituitary d.
Desferal
desferrioxamine mesylate
desipramine
desire
inhibited sexual d.
deslanoside
17,20-desmolase
20–22-desmolase
desmopressin
desmopressin acetate (DDAVP)
desmosome
desogestrel
3-keto d.
desoxycorticosterone
Desoxyn
desquamative inflammatory vaginitis
Desyrel
detachment
retinal d.
detection
d. bias
ectopic pregnancy d.
mammographic d.
prenatal d.
determinant
antigen d.
d. group
determination
blood gas d.
hemoglobin A_{Ic} d.
parentage d.
prenatal sex d.
sex d.
testis d.
Dethyrona
Dethyrone
detrusor
d. instability
d. muscle
developing fetus
development
abnormal fetal d.
CNS d.
early follicular d.
endometrial d.
excretory system d.
fetal d.
genital d.
goiter d.
male genital duct d.
mental d.
neurologic d.
reproductive system d.
developmental
d. age
d. diapause
Deventer's pelvis
deviation
standard d.

device
barium-impregnated plastic intrauterine d.
compression d.
contraceptive d.
Copper 7 intrauterine d.
copper intrauterine d.
Copper T intrauterine d.
corrective d.
intrauterine d. (IUD)
intrauterine contraceptive device (IUCD)
Lippes-type intrauterine d.
progesterone-releasing T-shaped d.
DeWees forceps
Dewey forceps
DEXA
dual-energy x-ray absorptiometry
Dex-A-Diet
dexamethasone
d. suppression test
Dexamfetamine
Dexatrim
dexbrompheniramine
dexchlorpheniramine
Dexedrine
Dexone
Dexon suture
dexpanthenol
dextran
high molecular weight d.
d. instillation
dextroamphetamine
dextro-norgestrel
dextrose
dextrothyroxine
dextroversion
dGMP
deoxyguanylic acid
DHE
dihydroergotamine
DHEA
dehydroepiandrosterone
DHEAS
dehydroepiandrosterone sulfate
DHT
dihydrotestosterone
diabetes
brittle d.
class A d.
gestational d. (GDM)
d. insipidus
insulin-dependent d. mellitus (IDDM)
maternal d.
d. mellitus
non-insulin-dependent d. mellitus (NIDDM)
overt insulin-dependent d. mellitus
poorly controlled maternal d.
type I d.
type II d.
diabetic
d. embryopathy
d. fetopathy
insulin-dependent d.
d. ketoacidosis
d. mother
d. nephropathy
d. pregnancy
pregnant d.
d. retinopathy
Diabinese
diacetate
ethynodiol d.
diacylglycerol
diagnosis
antenatal d.
colposcopic d.
early d.
fetal d.
genetic d.
histologic d.
histopathological d.
neonatal d.
prenatal d.
prenatal genetic d.
ultrasound d.
diagnostic
d. accuracy
d. imaging
d. model
d. procedure
d. radiation
diagonal conjugate
diakinesis
d. stage
Dialose
dialysis
kidney d.
peritoneal d.

diameter
anteroposterior d. of the pelvic inlet
Baudelocque's d.
biischial d.
biparietal d. (BPD)
bitemporal d.
conjugate d. of the pelvic inlet
fetal biparietal d.
gestational sac mean d.
intertuberous d.
d. medianus
d. obliqua
oblique d.
occipitofrontal d.
occipitomental d.
posterior sagittal d.
suboccipitobregmatic d.
trachelobregmatic d.
transverse d., d. transversa
diamine oxidase
cis-**diamminedichloroplatinum (DDP)**
cis-**diamminedichloroplatinum II**
diamniotic
Diamox
Dianabol
diapause
developmental d.
diaphanography
diaphragm
contraceptive d.
intrauterine d.
pelvic d.
d. pessary
urogenital d.
diaphragmatic hernia
Diapid
diarrhea
diastasis
d. recti
diastrophic dysplasia
diathermy
electrocoagulation d.
diatrizoate
diazepam
diazoxide
Dibenzyline
dibromodulcitol
dibromodulcitol with doxorubicin and vincristine (DAV)
DIC
disseminated intravascular coagulation
dichlorphenamide
dichorial, dichorionic
dicloxacillin sodium
dictyate stage
dicumarol
dicyclomine
didelphic uterus
didelphys
uterus d.
dienestrol
diet
high-fiber d.
low-residue d.
vegetarian d.
dietary
d. amenorrhea
d. fat
d. fiber
d. problem
diethylamide
lysergic acid d. (LSD)
diethylpropion
diethylstilbestrol (DES)
difference
arteriovenous oxygen d.
racial d.
differential
d. cell count
d. effect
d. vascular resistance
differentiation
central nervous system d.
fetal sexual d.
genital d.
male sex d.
sexual d.
testicular d.
diffuse fibrocystic disease
Diflucan
DiGeorge syndrome
digestive system
digitalis
digital radiography
digitoxin
digoxin
dihydrocodeine bitartrate
dihydrocodeinone
dihydroergotamine (DHE)
dihydroergotamine mesylate plus sodium heparin

dihydrofolate reductase inhibitor
dihydromorphinone hydrochloride
5α-dihydroprogesterone
20-α-dihydroprogestin dehydrogenase
dihydrotachysterol
dihydrotestosterone (DHT)
dihydroxyphenylalanine (dopa, DOPA, Dopa)
dihydroxyprogesterone acetophenide
1,25-dihydroxyvitamin D_3
diiodohydroxyquin
diiodohydroxyquinoline
diisopropyl fluorophosphate
Dilantin
dilated collateral vein
dilation, dilatation
  cervical d.
  d. and curettage (D & C)
  d. and evacuation (D & E)
  Frank technique of d.
dilator
  Goodell's d.
  Hanks d.'s
  Hegar's d.'s
  Lucite d.
  Pratt d.
  vaginal d.
  Walther's d.
Dilaudid
dildo, dildoe
Dimelor
dimenhydrinate
Dimetabs
Dimetane
dimethindene maleate
dimethothiazine mesylate
dimethyl-triazeno-imidazole carboxamide (DTIC)
dimethylxanthine
dimetria
dimidiate
dinitrate
  isosorbide d.
dinitrochlorobenzene
dinitrofluorobenzene
Diocto
Diodoquin
Dioeze
3α-diol-G
  5α-androstane-3α,17β-diol glucuronide
Diosuccin
Dio-Sul
Dioval
dioxide
  carbon d. (CO_2)
dioxin
dioxyline
dip
  type I d.
  type II d.
dipalmitoylphosphatidylcholine
diphemanil methylsulfate
diphenadione
Diphenadryl
Diphenatol
diphenhydramine
diphenoxylate hydrochloride
diphenylhydantoin
diphosphate
  menadiol sodium d.
diphosphate-choline
  cytidine d.-c.
diphosphate-diacylglycerol
  cytidine d.-d.
diphosphoglycerate
diploid distribution
dipyridamole
direct
  d. maternal death
  d. ovular transmigration
disability
  neurodevelopmental d.
Disalcid
disappearance
  fetal d.
disaturated
  d. lecithin
  d. phosphatidylcholine
discharge
  hospital d.
  d. instructions
  nipple d.
  pulsatile d.
  d. summary
  vaginal d.
discomfort
  breast d.
  pelvic d.
discoplacenta
discordancy
  growth d.
discordant artery flow velocity waveform
discus proligerus

disease
- ABO hemolytic d. of the newborn
- acute fatty liver d.
- Addison's d.
- adhesive d.
- adrenal gland d.
- allogeneic d.
- aortic valve d.
- arterial occlusive d.
- arterial vascular d.
- autoimmune d.
- benign breast d.
- Berger's renal d.
- breast d.
- cardiac d.
- cardiovascular d.
- cerebrovascular d.
- cholesterol ester storage d.
- Christmas d.
- chronic vascular d.
- collagen d.
- collagen-vascular d.
- congenital heart d.
- connective tissue d.
- coronary artery d.
- coronary heart d.
- Crohn's d.
- Cushing's d.
- cyanotic heart d.
- cystic d. of the breast
- cytomegalic inclusion d.
- diffuse fibrocystic d.
- distal tubal d.
- end-stage kidney d.
- Fabry's d.
- Farber's d.
- fetal heart d.
- fibrocystic d.
- fibrocystic d. of the breast
- Fox-Fordyce d.
- gallbladder d.
- Gaucher's d.
- genetic d.
- gestational trophoblastic d. (GTD)
- glycogen-storage d.
- Graves' d.
- Hansen's d.
- Hartnup d.
- heart d.
- hemoglobin C d.
- hemoglobin H d.
- hemolytic d. of the newborn
- Hodgkin's d.
- homologous d.
- Huntington's d.
- hyaline membrane d. of the newborn
- hypothalamic d.
- I-cell d.
- inflammatory bowel d.
- intraperitoneal endometrial metastatic d.
- ischemic heart d.
- kidney d.
- Krabbe's d.
- kyphoscoliotic heart d.
- Legionnaires' d.
- liver d.
- Lyme d.
- maple syrup urine d.
- maternal d.
- maternal cyanotic heart d.
- Minamata d.
- mixed connective-tissue d.
- Mondor's d.
- neoplastic trophoblastic d.
- New York Heart Association classification of heart d.
- Nicolas-Favre d.
- Niemann-Pick d.
- oxygen toxicity lung d.
- Paget's d.
- parathyroid d.
- Parkinson's d.
- pelvic inflammatory d. (PID)
- peptic ulcer d.
- pituitary d.
- placental-site gestational trophoblastic d.
- polycystic kidney d.
- polycystic ovarian d.
- polycystic renal d.
- postpartum pleuropulmonary and cardiac d.
- preinvasive cervical d.
- premalignant d.
- psychosomatic d.
- pulmonary d.
- renal d.
- Rh d.
- rheumatic d.

rheumatic heart d.
Rh hemolytic d.
Ritter's d.
runt d.
Sandhoff's d.
SC d.
sclerocystic d. of the ovary
secretory d.
sexually transmitted d. (STD)
sickle cell d.
sickle cell-hemoglobin C d. (S-C disease)
sickle cell-hemoglobin D d. (S-D disease)
sickle cell-hemoglobin S d.
sickle cell-thalassemia d.
sickle cell-β-thalassemia d.
silent pelvic inflammatory d.
Simmonds' d.
sixth d.
skin d.
Still's d.
Tay-Sachs d.
thromboembolic d. (TE)
thyroid d.
thyroid gland d.
trophoblastic d.
trophoblastic neoplastic d.
tubulointerstitial d.
underlying renal d.
valvular heart d.
vascular d.
venereal d.
von Recklinghausen's d.
von Willebrand's d.
Wilson's d.
Wolman's d.
X-linked dominant d.
X-linked recessive d.

disengagement
disgerminoma
Disipal
disk, disc
d. abnormality
embryonic d.
dislocation
congenital hip d.
hip d.
disodium
etidronate d.
intermittent cyclical etidronate d.
Disonate
disopyramide
disorder
affective d.
arrest d.
autosomal d.
autosomal chromosome d.
autosomal dominant d.
autosomal recessive d.
brain d.
cardiopulmonary d.
coagulation d.
connective tissue d.
eating d.
emotional d.
endocrine d.
gastrointestinal d.
genetic d.
hematologic d.
hematopoietic d.
heme metabolism d.
hepatic d.
hypothalamic-pituitary d.
inherited d.
lysosomal enzyme d.
mendelian d.
metabolic d.
metal metabolism d.
musculoskeletal d.
neurologic d.
ovarian d.
parathyroid d.
pelvic support d.
pituitary d.
platelet d.
polygenic d.
porphyrin metabolism d.
psychiatric d.
pulmonary d.
purine metabolism d.
recessive d.
reproductive d.
rheumatologic d.
seizure d.
transport d.
urinary tract d.
X-linked d.
disperse placenta
disproportion
cephalopelvic d.
fetopelvic d.

disputed maternity
disruption
anal sphincter d.
perineal d.
perineal sphincter d.
dissecting aortic aneurysm
dissection
groin d.
inguinal-femoral node d.
pelvic node d.
selective inguinal node d.
disseminated
d. gonococcal infection
d. gonorrhea
d. infection
d. intravascular coagulation (DIC)
dissemination
iatrogenic d.
dissociation constant
distal
d. occlusion
d. tubal disease
d. tubal microsurgery
d. tubal obstruction
distance
source axis d. (SAD)
source-to-skin d. (SSD)
distention
abdominal d.
distigmine bromide
distress
fetal d.
iatrogenic fetal d.
neonatal d.
respiratory d.
transient fetal d.
distribution
depth-dose d.
diploid d.
tetraploid d.
disturbance
architectural d.
mental d.
ovulatory d.
visual d.
disulfiram
Ditropan
Diucardin
Diuchlor H
Diulo
Diurese-R
diuresis
diuretic
thiazide d.
Diuril
diversion
urinary d.
diverticulitis
diverticulum, pl. **diverticula**
tubal d.
urethral d.
diverting colostomy
division
cellular d.
premature centromere d.
transcervical d.
divorce
d. counseling
separation and d.
DMPA
demedroxyprogesterone acetate
DNA
deoxyribonucleic acid
DNA amplification
complementary DNA (cDNA)
DNA hybridization
DNA index
DNA marker
DNA sequence
Y-specific DNA
DOAK Tar
dobutamine
Dobutrex
DOC
deoxycorticosterone
docusate
d. calcium
d. sodium
Döhle body
Doktors
Dolacet
Dolanex
Dolene
dolichocephalic head
dolichopellic, dolichopelvic
Dolophine
domestic violence
dominance
thromboxane d.
dominant
d. follicle
d. inheritance
donation
autologous blood d.

embryo d.
oocyte d.
sperm d.
donor
artificial insemination d. (AID)
d. sperm
Donovan body
donovanosis
donut pessary
dopa, DOPA, Dopa
dihydroxyphenylalanine
L-dopa
levodopa
Dopamet
dopamine
d. agonist
d. receptor agonist
dopaminergic agonist
Dopar
Doppler
D. effect
D. evaluation
D. flow
D. flow-velocity wave form
D. principle
D. shift
D. ultrasonography
D. ultrasound
D. velocimetry
D. waveform
dorsal birthing position
dosage
dose
average radiation d.
central axis depth d.
depth d.
maximal permissible d.
minimum lethal d. (MLD)
physiologic replacement d.
radiation d.
Doss
dot-blot procedure
dothiepin
double
d. bubble sign
d. cell (D cell)
d. gloving
d. helix
d. J stent
d. ureter
double-balloon catheter
double-freeze technique
double-mouthed uterus
double-tooth tenaculum
doubling time
douche
douching
iodine d.
maternal d.
povidone-iodine d.
vaginal d.
Douglas'
D. cul-de-sac
D. mechanism
D. pouch
D. spontaneous evolution
down regulation
Down's syndrome
doxepin
doxorubicin
Doxy-Caps
doxycycline
doxylamine
Doyle's operation
D^u-positive mother
dragging
drain
Penrose d.
retroperitoneal d.
drainage
hematoma d.
lymphatic d.
lymph node d.
percutaneous d.
suction d.
Dramamine
Dramilin
Dramocen
Dramoject
dressing forceps
Drew-Smythe catheter
Dripps–American Society of Anesthesiologists classification
Drisdol
Drize
droperidol
drug
acne d.
d. addiction
adrenergic d.
anticholinergic d.
anticonvulsant d.
antihypertensive d.
antimalarial d.
antineoplastic d.

drug *(continued)*
antipsychotic d.
antithyroid d.
beta-adrenergic d.
cholinergic d.
hypertensive d.
intravenous d.
nonestrogen d.
nonsteroidal anti-inflammatory d. (NSAID)
d. prescription
psychiatric d.
psychoactive d.
psychotropic d.
recreational d.
social d.
d. use counseling
drug-depressed infant
drug-induced fever
dry labor
DTIC
dimethyl-triazeno-imidazole carboxamide
DTIC-Dome
dTMP
deoxythymidylic acid
dual-energy x-ray absorptiometry (DEXA)
DUB
dysfunctional uterine bleeding
Dubowitz score
Duchenne's
D. muscular dystrophy
D. paralysis
duckbill speculum
duct
Bartholin's d.
focally dilated d.
Gartner's d.
genital d.
lactiferous d.
male genital d.
mesonephric d.
metanephric d.
müllerian d.
d. papilloma
paramesonephric d.
paraurethral d.
Skene's d.
solitary dilated d.
vestibular d.
wolffian d.
ductal
d. adenoma
d. carcinoma
d. ectasia
d. hyperplasia
ductule
ductus
d. arteriosus
d. venosus
Dührssen's
D. incisions
Dukes classification
Dumontpallier's pessary
Duncan's
D. curette
D. folds
D. mechanism of placental delivery
Duosol
Duotrate
Duphalac
duplex
d. ultrasound
d. uterus
duplication
gene d.
duplicitas
d. anterior
Duracillin AS
Dura-Estrin
Duragen
dural spinal angioma
Duraquin
Duretic
dust
angel d.
Dutch cap
duty
breach of d.
d. cycle
negligence of d.
Duvoid
DVT
deep venous thrombosis
dwarf
d. pelvis
d. syndrome
dwarfism
lethal d.
Dycill
Dyflos
dying
Dymelor

Dymenate
dynamics
androgen d.
dynamic test of hormone level
Dynapen
dynorphin
Dynothel
dyphylline
Dyrenium
dyschezia
dysentery
dysfibrinogenemia
dysfunction
associated d.
bladder d.
cerebral d.
corpus luteum d.
hypertonic uterine d.
hypothalamic d.
hypothalamic-pituitary d.
hypotonic uterine d.
lymphocyte d.
postoperative bladder d.
postoperative voiding d.
sexual d.
thyroid d.
urinary bladder d.
uterine d.
voiding d.
dysfunctional
d. labor pattern
d. uterine bleeding (DUB)
dysgenesis
gonadal d.
mixed gonadal d.
ovarian d.
pure gonadal d.
renal d.
X-linked recessive XY gonadal d.
XY gonadal d.
dysgerminoma
ovarian d.
dysmature
dysmaturity
d. syndrome
dysmenorrhea
essential d.
functional d.
intrinsic d.
mechanical d.
membranous d.
obstructive d.
ovarian d.
primary d.
secondary d.
spasmodic d.
tubal d.
ureteral d.
uterine d.
vaginal d.
dysmenorrheal membrane
dysmorphology
dysontogenetic cyst
dyspareunia
dysplasia
bronchopulmonary d.
cervical d.
chondroectodermal d.
diastrophic d.
ectodermal d.
fetal skeletal d.
high-grade cervical d.
intraepithelial cervical d.
mammary d.
polycystic fibrous d.
polyostotic fibrous d.
radiation d.
skeletal d.
thanatophoric d.
dyspnea
dysrhythmia
cardiac d.
gastric d.
dystocia
fetal d.
maternal d.
placental d.
shoulder d.
dystrophic calcification
dystrophy
Duchenne's muscular d.
muscular d.
myotonic d.
short-limb d.
vulvar d.
dysuria
dysuria-sterile pyuria syndrome

E

E_2
estradiol
EACA
epsilon-aminocaproic acid
ε-aminocaproic acid
early
e. ambulation
e. cardiac motion
e. deceleration
e. diagnosis
e. drug use
e. embryonic death
e. embryonic loss
e. follicular development
e. neonatal death
e. organogenesis
e. pregnancy factor
e. pregnancy loss
e. pregnancy test
e. pregnancy wastage
e. stromal invasion
e. vulvar carcinoma
early-onset preeclampsia
eating
e. disorder
e. habits
Ebstein's anomaly
eccrine gland
eccyesis
ECG
electrocardiogram
echinococcal cyst
echinocyte
echo
e. formation
scattered e.
specular e.
echocardiography
echogenic tissue
echothiophate iodide
echovirus
eclampsia
puerperal e.
superimposed e.
eclamptic
e. retinopathy
e. seizure
eclamptogenic, eclamptogenous
Ecotrin
ectasia, ectasis
ductal e.
mammary duct e.
ectocervical
ectocervix
ectoderm
ectodermal dysplasia
ectoparasite
ectopic
e. decidua
e. endometrial tissue
e. pregnancy
e. pregnancy detection
e. pregnancy rate
e. pregnancy reimplantation
e. ureter
ectropion
cervical e.
congenital e.
EDC
estimated/expected date of confinement
estimated date of conception
Edecrin
edema
cerebral e.
gestational e.
leg e.
lung e.
menstrual e.
e. neonatorum
premenstrual e.
pulmonary e.
vulvar e.
edrophonium chloride
education
patient e.
Edwards' syndrome
EEG
electroencephalogram
effacement
cervical e.
effect
adverse e.
adverse drug e.
anemic e.
antiestrogenic e.
Arias-Stella e.
Bohr e.
cardiovascular e.

effect *(continued)*
Compton e.
cytotoxic e.
differential e.
Doppler e.
estrogen e.
hormonal e.
hypnotic e.
Mach band e.
marijuana e.
neurologic adverse e.
oral e.
perinatal e.
pituitary gonadotropin e.
possible teratogenic e.
psychological e.
sedative e.
social factor e.
star e.
teratogenic e.
effective
e. conjugate
e. period
effector cell
efficacy
oral contraceptive e.
efficiency
female fertility e.
effluvium
telogen e.
Effortil
effusion
malignant e.
malignant pleural e.
pleural e.
Efroxine
Efudex
EGF
epidermal growth factor
egg
e. transport
e. vestment
e. yolk extender
EH
endometrial hyperplasia
Ehlers-Danlos syndrome
EIC
extensive intraductal component
eicosanoid
eight-cell embryo
EIN
endometrial intraepithelial neoplasia
Eisenmenger syndrome
ejaculate
ejaculation
ejecta
laser e.
ejection
milk e.
Eklund technique
elastic stocking
Elavil
elderly
e. primigravida
electricity
electrocardiogram (ECG)
electrocardiography
fetal e.
electrocautery
laparoscopic e.
transurethral e.
electrocoagulation diathermy
electrode
spiral e.
electroencephalogram (EEG)
electrohysterograph
electrolysis
electrolyte
e. imbalance
electromagnetic
e. radiation
e. spectrum
electromyography
electron
electronic
e. fetal monitor
e. fetal monitoring
electron-volt (eV, ev)
electroshock therapy
elephantiasis
e. vulvae
elevated
e. enzyme activity
e. liver enzymes
elevation
alpha-fetoprotein e.
fetus growth e.
ELISA
enzyme-linked immunosorbent assay
Elixicon
Elixomin
Elixophyllin
Elliot forceps
Ellis-van Creveld syndrome

elongation
Eltroxin
Embolex
embolism
amniotic fluid e.
cerebral e.
pulmonary e.
embolization
e. therapy
transcatheter e.
embolus, pl. **emboli**
amniotic fluid e.
gas e.
Gianturco spring e.
pulmonary emboli
trophoblastic e.
embryatrics
embryo
abnormal e.
e. donation
eight-cell e.
four-cell e.
e. reduction
e. transfer
e. visualization
embryogenesis
embryology
breast e.
genital tract e.
Leydig cell e.
reproductive tract e.
embryonal
e. carcinoma
e. rhabdomyosarcoma
embryonic
e. cleavage
e. disk
e. loss
e. period
embryonization
embryopathy
diabetic e.
embryoscopy
embryotomy
eminence
median e.
Emko
emmenagogic
emmenagogue
emmenia
emmenic
emmeniopathy
emmenology
Emmet's operation
emotional
e. amenorrhea
e. disorder
e. stress
emphysema
Empirin
empty
e. scrotum syndrome
e. sella syndrome
enalapril
enanthate
estradiol e.
norethindrone e. (NET-EN)
en bloc resection
encainide
encapsulation
Encare
encephalitis
HSV-1 e.
HSV-2 e.
neonatal HSV-1 e.
neonatal HSV-2 e.
encephalocele
encephalopathy
hypertensive e.
hypoxic ischemic e.
neonatal e.
newborn hypoxic ischemic e.
Endep
endocardial fibroelastosis
endocarditis
bacterial e.
infective e.
endocervical
e. canal
e. canal colposcopy
e. canal curettage
e. curettage
e. mucosa
e. polyp
e. sampling brush
endocervicitis
endocervix
endochondroma
endocolpitis
endocrine
e. disorder
e. factor
e. gland
e. system
e. test

endocrinology
reproductive e.
endocytosis
receptor-mediated e.
endoderm
endodermal sinus tumor
endodermatosis
endogenous
e. catecholamine
e. estrogen
e. estrogen level
e. gonadotropin activity suppression
e. hormone
e. opiate
e. opiate receptor
e. opioid peptide
e. pyrogen
e. steroid
endometrial
e. ablation
e. adenoacanthoma
e. adenocarcinoma
e. adenosquamous carcinoma
e. atrophy
e. biopsy
e. breakdown
e. cancer
e. carcinoma
e. clear cell adenocarcinoma
e. cycle
e. cycling activity
e. cyst
e. development
e. histology
e. hyperplasia (EH)
e. implant
e. intraepithelial neoplasia (EIN)
e. metastasizing leiomyoma
e. morphology
e. neoplasia
e. polyp
e. protein
e. receptor
e. resection
e. sampling
e. sarcoma
e. secretory adenocarcinoma
e. spiral artery
e. stimulation
e. stromal sarcoma (ESS)
e. thickness
e. tuberculosis
endometrioid
e. carcinoma
e. tumor
endometrioma
large e.
endometriosis
American Fertility Society classification of e.
asymptomatic mild e.
e. interna
internal e.
mild e.
ovarian e.
rectosigmoid colon e.
retroperitoneal e.
severe e.
small bowel e.
tubal e.
urinary tract e.
vulvar e.
endometriosis-associated infertility
endometriotic focus
endometritis
decidual e.
e. dissecans
endometrium, pl. **endometria**
cyclic proliferative e.
decidualized e.
inactive e.
menstrual e.
nonpregnant e.
e. sampling
Swiss cheese e.
tubal e.
endometropic
endomyometritis
endonuclease
restriction e.
endoparametritis
endopelvic fascia
endophytic
endorphin
endorphin, dopamine, and prostaglandin theory
endosalpingiosis
endosalpingitis
endosalpingoblastosis
endoscopic
e. retrograde cholangiopancreatography
e. visualization

endoscopy
colorectal cancer e.
endothelial cell
endothelin plasma level
endotheliochorial placenta
endothelio-endothelial placenta
endotheliosis
glomerular capillary e.
endotoxin
endotracheal
e. intubation
e. tube
endotrachelitis
endovaginal
e. finding
e. probe
endovasculitis
hemorrhagic e.
end-stage kidney disease
Enduron
enema
barium e.
Cort e.
energy expenditure
enflurane
engagement
English
E. lock
E. position
engorged breast
engorgement
breast e.
vascular e.
engraftment
fetal e.
enhancement
e. factor
immunologic e.
Enkaid
enkephalin
enlargement
abdominal e.
adenomyosis in uterine e.
clitoris e.
parotid e.
pelvis e.
sellar e.
Enovid
Entamoeba histolytica
enteritis
regional e.
Enterobacter
Enterobius vermicularis
enterocele
enterococcus, pl. **enterococci**
enterocolitis
necrotizing e.
pseudomembranous e.
enteromenia
enterotoxin F
enterovaginal fistula
Enterovirus
environment
work e.
environmental toxin
enzyme
e. activity
e. assay
e. deficiency
elevated liver e.'s
e. immunoassay
proteolytic e.
enzyme-linked
e.-l. antiglobulin testing
e.-l. immunosorbent assay (ELISA)
enzymopathy
eosinophilia
EP
etoposide
EPC
external pneumatic calf compression
ephedrine
e. sulfate
epidemic
epidemiological
e. characteristic
e. feature
epidemiology
epidermal
e. growth factor (EGF)
e. growth factor-like growth factor
e. inclusion cyst
epidermoid carcinoma
epidermolysis
e. bullosa
epididymal sperm
epidural
e. analgesia
e. anesthesia
e. hemangioma
e. morphine
Epifrin

epigastric
e. artery
e. hernia
e. pain
e. spigelian hernia
epilepsy
e. management
epimenorrhagia
epimenorrhea
Epinal
epinephrine
epiphyseal ossification center
episioperineorrhaphy
episioplasty
episiorrhaphy
episiostenosis
episiotomy
median e.
mediolateral e.
primarily resutured e.
ruptured e.
17-epitestosterone
epithelial
e. autoantibody localization
e. cancer
e. cyst
e. hyperplasia
e. ovarian carcinoma
e. stromal ovarian neoplasm
e. stromal tumor
e. tumor
epitheliochorial placenta
epithelium
aceto-white e.
atypical e.
cervical e.
coelomic e.
columnar e.
germinal e.
native squamous e.
ovarian germinal e.
papilla of columnar e.
squamous e.
stratified squamous e.
surface e.
uterine e.
white e.
Epo
erythropoietin
epoophorectomy
epoophoron
Eppendorf punch biopsy forceps
Eppy/N
Eprolin
epsilon-aminocaproic acid, ε-aminocaproic acid (EACA)
epulis
e. gravidarum
e. of pregnancy
Equagesic
Equanil
equation
Henderson-Hasselbalch e.
Kučera's e.
equilibrium
acid-base e.
equinovarus
talipes e.
Erb's palsy
ergocalciferol
ergonovine
e. maleate
ergot
ergotamine
e. tartrate
Ergotrate
erigentes
nervi e.
erosion
cervical e.
erosive adenomatosis of nipple
error
alpha e.
beta e.
metabolic e.
erysipelas
e. internum
erythema
e. chronicum migrans
e. infectiosum
e. neonatorum
e. nodosum
palmar e.
e. toxicum neonatorum
erythematosus
lupus e. (LE)
systemic lupus e. (SLE)
erythrityl tetranitrate
erythroblastosis fetalis
Erythrocin
erythrocyte
e. count
e. enzyme deficiency
e. membrane
packed e.

e. sedimentation rate
e. transfusion
erythrocytosis
Erythromid
erythromycin
e. therapy
erythron
erythroplasia
Zoon's e.
erythropoiesis
erythropoietin (Epo)
Escherichia
E. coli
E. coli vaccine
escutcheon
Eserine
Esidrix
Eskalith
esmolol hydrochloride
esophageal
e. atresia
e. varices
esophagitis
reflux e.
esophagus
ESS
endometrial stromal sarcoma
essential dysmenorrhea
Estes
E. operation
E. procedure
estetrol
esthiomene
estimated
e. date of conception (EDC)
estimated/expected date of confinement (EDC)
estimation
gestational age e.
estradiol (E_2)
e. assay
e. blood level
bound e.
e. cypionate
e. enanthate
ethinyl e.
free e.
e. 2-hydroxylation
micronized e.
e. receptor
e. suppression
e. valerate
estradiol-17β
17β-estradiol
17β-e. dehydrogenase
estrane
Estratab
Estratest
Estraval
estriol
e. level
Estro-Cyp
estrogen
e. breakthrough bleeding
catechol e.
conjugated e.'s
conjugated equine e.
e. deprivation
e. effect
endogenous e.
e. excess
e. level
e. loss
e. metabolism
oral conjugated e.
orally administered e.
postcoital e.
e. receptor
e. receptor localization
e. replacement
e. replacement therapy
serum e.
e. sulfotransferase
e. surge
e. synthesis
e. therapy
uninterrupted e.
unopposed e.
e. use
e. window etiologic hypothesis
e. withdrawal
e. withdrawal bleeding
estrogen-assisted colposcopy
estrogen-induced prolactinoma
estrogen/progesterone ratio
estrogen-progesterone withdrawal bleeding
estrogen-progestin
e.-p. artificial cycle
e.-p. contraceptive
e.-p. replacement therapy
e.-p. test
estrogen-progestogen combination
Estroject

estrone
oral e.
estrus
ethacrynic acid
ethambutol hydrochloride
Ethamide
ethanol
ethchlorvynol
ether
ethical
e. issue
e. standard
ethics
medical e.
ethinamate
ethinyl estradiol
ethinyl testosterone
ethiodized oil
Ethiodol
ethionamide
ethisterone
ethnicity
ethoheptazine citrate
ethopropazine hydrochloride
ethosuximide
ethotoin
ethoxzolamide
Ethrane
ethyl biscoumacetate
ethylnorepinephrine
ethylphenylephrine
ethynodiol
e. diacetate
ethynyl, ethinyl
Etibi
etidronate disodium
etiocholanolone
etiology
etoposide (EP)
etretinate
Eubacterium
eugonadotropic
e. amenorrhea
e. hypogonadism
eukaryote
Eulipos
euploid abortion
euprolactinemic woman
Euthroid
Eutonyl
eV, ev
electron-volt
evacuation
fimbrial e.
evaluation
Doppler e.
infertility e.
mental status e.
urological e.
uterine e.
evaporation
event
iatrogenic e.
life e.
Everard Williams procedure
eversion
cervical e.
evidence
rape e.
evisceration
evoked potential technique
evolution
Denman's spontaneous e.
Douglas' spontaneous e.
spontaneous e.
Ewing's sarcoma
exaggerated craniocaudal view
examination
abdominal e.
bimanual pelvic e.
chest e.
dark-field e.
eye e.
neonate e.
neurologic e.
newborn e.
pelvic e.
physical e.
radiological e.
rectal e.
rectovaginal e.
self-breast e.
speculum e.
stool e.
vaginal e.
excess
androgen e.
estrogen e.
soluble antigen e.
excessive blood loss
exchange
e. transfusion
e. transfusion treatment
excision
e. biopsy

local e.
radical e.
excitation
excretion
sodium e.
water e.
excretory system development
exenteration
anterior e.
anterior pelvic e.
pelvic e.
posterior pelvic e.
pyelonephritis in e.
stress reaction in e.
total e.
total pelvic e.
exercise
Kegel's e.'s
maternal e.
pelvic e.
exhaustion
ovarian follicle e.
Exna
exocelomic membrane
exocervix
exocytosis
exogenous
e. gonadotropin
e. gonadotropin stimulation
e. hormone
e. human menopausal gonadotropin
e. sex hormone
exophytic
exostosis
pelvic e.
exotoxin
e. C
Pseudomonas e.
expansion
plasma volume e.
volume e.
expectancy
life e.
expectant management
expenditure
energy e.
experience
sexual e.
expert witness
exploratory laparotomy
exposure
anesthetic gas e.
DES e.
maternal mercury e.
methamphetamine e.
prenatal diethylstilbestrol e.
expressivity
expulsion
expulsive
e. force
e. pains
extended
e. field irradiation therapy
e. radical mastectomy
e. rubella syndrome
extender
egg yolk e.
extension
extensive intraductal component (EIC)
external
e. beam irradiation
e. cephalic version
e. conjugate
e. genitalia
e. hemorrhage
e. os
e. ovular transmigration
e. pneumatic calf compression (EPC)
e. radiation therapy
e. rotation
e. version
e. x-ray therapy
extraamniotic pregnancy
extracellular fluid
extrachorial pregnancy
extracorporeal membrane oxygenation
extract
extraction
breech e.
menstrual e.
podalic e.
vacuum e.
extractor
Bird's vacuum e.
Kobayashi vacuum e.
Malmström vacuum e.
Mityvac vacuum e.
Murless head e.
plastic cup vacuum e.
Silastic cup e.
vacuum e.

extradural
e. anesthesia
e. block
extraembryonic fetal membrane
extrafascial hysterectomy
extraglandular
e. conversion
e. estrogen production
extramedullary hematopoiesis
extramembranous pregnancy
extraovular
extrapelvic malignancy
extraperitoneal cesarean section
extrauterine pregnancy
extremity
lower e.
extrusion
oocyte e.
placental e.
extubation

F

Fabricius
bursa of F.
Fabry's disease
face presentation
facial
f. nerve
f. nerve palsy
f. nerve paralysis
f. paralysis
facies
F.A.C.O.G.
Fellow of the American College of Obstetricians and Gynecologists
FACS
fluorescent-activated cell sorter
factitious precocious puberty
factor
f. VIII
f. VIII:C
f. Xa
acidic fibroblast growth f. (FGFa)
alloimmune f.
angiogenic growth f.
autoimmune f.
blocking f.
cervical f.
chemotactic f.
citrovorum f.
coagulation f.
coital f.
colony-stimulating f.
f. concentrate
corticotropin-releasing f.
cytotoxic f.
f. II deficiency
f. V deficiency
f. VII deficiency
f. IX deficiency
f. X deficiency
f. XI deficiency
f. XIII deficiency
early pregnancy f.
endocrine f.
enhancement f.
epidermal growth f. (EGF)
epidermal growth factor-like growth f.
fetal f.
fibroblast growth f.
fibroblast pneumocyte f.
follicular f.
granulocyte colony-stimulating f. (G-CSF)
granulocyte-macrophage colony-stimulating f. (GM-CSF)
growth f. (GF)
growth-like f.
helper f.
HG f.
humoral f.
immune f.
infertility f.
f. VII inhibitor
insulin-like growth f. (IGF)
kidney-derived growth f.
lymphocyte-activating f.
macrophage-activating f. (MAF)
macrophage colony-stimulating f.
macrophage-inhibition f.
male f.
maternal f.
microbial f.
migration-inhibitory f. (MIF)
mixed lymphocyte reaction blocking f.
mortality risk f.
müllerian duct inhibitory f.
obstetrical risk f.
ovarian f.
perinatal risk f.
platelet-activating f.
platelet-derived growth f.
prenatal risk f.
prognostic f.
prolactin inhibiting f. (PIF)
prolactin releasing f. (PRF)
Rh f.
Rh-negative f.
risk f.
social f.
testes-determining f.
transfer f.
transforming growth f.
tubal f.
tumor angiogenesis f. (TAF)

factor *(continued)*
tumor-limiting f.
tumor necrosis f. (TNF)
uterine f.
factor-α
tumor necrosis f.-α
failed forceps
failure
acute renal f.
bone marrow f.
cardiac f.
congestive heart f.
contraceptive f.
fertility f.
fimbrial f.
gonadal f.
heart f.
hypothalamic f.
implantation f.
kidney f.
multiple organ f.
ovarian f.
premature ovarian f.
primary ovarian f.
renal f.
reproductive f.
f. to thrive
falling of the womb
fallopian
f. pregnancy
f. tube
f. tube carcinoma
f. tube mass
f. tube metastasis
Fallot
tetralogy of F.
Falope ring
false
f. conjugate
f. knots
f. knots of umbilical cord
f. labor
f. mole
f. pains
f. pregnancy
f. waters
familial
f. cholesterolemia
f. hirsutism
f. hypercholesterolemia
f. hypofibrinogenemia
f. infertility
f. lipoid adrenal hyperplasia
f. tendency
family
f. history
f. physician
f. planning
Fanconi's
F. anemia
F. syndrome
Fansidar
faradism
Farber's disease
fascia
f. of breast
endopelvic f.
obturator f.
perirectal f.
subserous f.
fascial
f. necrosis
f. sling procedure
f. strip
fasciitis
necrotizing f.
Fastin
fasting
fast neutron
fat
f. density
dietary f.
f. flap
f. metabolism
f. necrosis
unsaturated f.
fatigue
fatty
f. halo
f. infiltration
f. liver of pregnancy
fatty acid-coenzyme A
fear
pregnancy f.
feature
epidemiological f.
fecal
f. diversion colostomy
f. impaction
fecund
fecundability
fecundate
fecundation
fecundity

Federation of Gynecology and Obstetrics classification
feeding
breast f.
Fellow of the American College of Obstetricians and Gynecologists (F.A.C.O.G.)
Felty's syndrome
female
f. catheter
f. fertility efficiency
f. fertility inefficiency
f. genital tract
f. hyperandrogenism screening
f. pseudohermaphroditism
f. puberty
f. reproductive tract
f. sterility
f. sterilization
f. urethra
feminization
incomplete testicular f.
f. syndrome
testicular f.
Feminone
Femogen Forte
Femogex
femoral
f. arterial catheter
f. artery catheterization
f. circumflex artery
f. hernia
f. lymph node
f. nerve
f. neuropathy
f. node
femur
f. length
fenamate
fenestration
laparoscopic f.
fenfluramine
fenoterol
fentanyl citrate
Fe_3O_4
magnetite
Ferguson reflex
ferning
f. technique
fern test
ferric sulfate
Ferriman and Gallwey hirsutism scoring system
ferritin
ferrous sulfate
fertile
f. period
f. phase
fertility
f. cycle
f. failure
male f.
f. rate
subsequent f.
fertilizable life span
fertilization
f. age
in vitro f.
in vivo f.
fertilized ovum
fetal
f. abdomen
f. abdominal abnormality
f. abdominal circumference
f. abnormality
f. acid-base balance
f. acid-base status
f. acidemia
f. acidosis
f. acoustic stimulation test
f. activity
f. activity test
f. adrenal gland
f. adrenocorticotropic hormone
f. age
f. alcohol syndrome
f. allograft survival
f. anatomy
f. anomaly
f. aorta
f. arrhythmia
f. asphyxia
f. aspiration syndrome
f. attitude
f. biparietal diameter
f. blood
f. blood flow
f. blood gas
f. blood glucose
f. blood oxygen-carrying capacity
f. blood pH
f. blood sampling

fetal *(continued)*
f. blood study
f. blood value
f. blood velocity
f. blood volume
f. body movement
f. bradycardia
f. brain
f. brain death
f. breathing
f. cardiac function
f. cardiac motion
f. cardiac output
f. cardiovascular system
f. cell
f. cellular growth
f. central nervous system abnormality
f. circulation
f. condition
f. congenital hyperplasia
f. cortisol infusion
f. cotyledon
f. cranial artery
f. cystic fibrosis
f. death
f. death rate
f. descent
f. development
f. diagnosis
f. disappearance
f. distress
f. dose limit
f. drug therapy
f. dystocia
f. electrocardiography
f. engraftment
f. factor
f. fracture
f. genital tract
f. genital tract tumor
f. growth
f. growth measurement
f. growth retardation
f. habitus
f. head
f. head:abdominal circumference ratio
f. head position
f. health
f. heart
f. heart action
f. heart disease
f. heart rate (FHR)
f. heart rate deceleration
f. heart rate monitoring
f. heart rate pattern
f. heart rate reactivity
f. heart rate variability
f. heart sound
f. hemodynamics
f. hemoglobin
f. hemorrhage
f. hormone
f. hydantoin syndrome
f. hydrops
f. hypoxia
f. imaging
f. infection
f. intracranial anatomy
f. jeopardy
f. karyotype
f. LDL level
f. lie
f. life
f. limb
f. liver
f. liver tumor
f. lung maturation
f. lung maturity
f. maceration
f. macrosomia
f. malformation
f. maturity
f. medicine
f. membrane
f. metabolism
f. monitoring
f. morbidity
f. mortality
f. movement
f. nutrition
f. outcome
f. outline
f. ovarian cyst
f. oxygenation
f. phenytoin syndrome
f. physiologist
f. position
f. postural abnormality
f. posture
f. presentation
f. pulmonary maturity
f. reduction
f. rejection
f. resorption

f. retention
f. risk
f. scalp blood sampling
f. scalp oxygenation
f. serum
f. sexual differentiation
f. skeletal dysplasia
f. skin sampling
f. skull depression
f. souffle
f. spine
f. squama, pl. squamae
f. station
f. steroid concentration
f. surgery
f. surveillance
f. swallowing
f. tachycardia
f. thoracic abnormality
f. thrombocytopenia
f. thyroid hormone
f. toxoplasmosis
f. transfusion
f. trauma
f. trimethadione syndrome
f. tumor
f. ultrasound
f. urinary tract
f. urination
f. uropathy
f. vascular anomaly
f. viability
f. warfarin syndrome
f. wastage
f. weight
f. well-being

fetalis
maternal hydrops f.
maternal Parvovirus f.

fetalism

fetal-maternal
f.-m. communication
f.-m. hemorrhage

fetal-neonatal transition

fetal-placental
f.-p. steroidogenesis
f.-p. unit

fetation

feticide

feto-fetal transfusion syndrome

fetography

fetology

fetometry
ultrasound f.

fetopathy
diabetic f.

fetopelvic disproportion

fetoplacental
f. access
f. anasarca
f. circulation
f. function

fetoprotein

fetoscope

fetoscopy

fetus, pl. **fetuses**
coexistent f.
f. compressus
developing f.
f. in fetu
f. growth elevation
growth-retarded f.
harlequin f.
HLA-compatible f.
impacted f.
nonstressed f.
f. papyraceus
previable f.
stressed f.
triploid f.

Feulgen stain

fever
absorption f.
childbed f.
drug-induced f.
milk f.
puerperal f.
rheumatic f.
scarlet f.
typhoid f.

FFP
fresh frozen plasma

FGFa
acidic fibroblast growth factor

FHR
fetal heart rate

FIA
fluorometric immunoassay

fiber
Dacron f.
dietary f.

fibrillation
atrial f.

fibrin
f. degradation product
f. sheath
fibrinogen
f. abnormality
plasma f.
fibrinogen-fibrin conversion syndrome
fibrinoid
fibrinolysis
fibrinolytic
f. agent
f. and clotting system
fibrinous polyp
fibroadenolipoma
degenerated f.
fibroadenoma
giant f.
intracanalicular f.
pericanalicular f.
fibroblast
f. growth factor
f. pneumocyte factor
fibrocystic
f. breast change
f. change
f. disease
f. disease of the breast
fibroelastosis
endocardial f.
fibroid
uterine f.
fibroidectomy
fibroma
f. molle gravidarum
ovarian f.
vulvar f.
fibromatosis
pelvic f.
fibromectomy
fibromuscular cervical stroma
fibromyoma of uterus
fibronectin
fibroplasia
retrolental f.
fibrosarcoma
fibrosing
f. adenomatosis
f. adenosis
fibrosis
cystic f.
fetal cystic f.
focal f.
horseshoe f.
postradiation periureteral f.
fibrous connective tissue
Fick principle
field
f. defect
visual f.
FIGO
International Federation of Gynecology and Obstetrics
F. nomenclature
figure
mitotic f.
filament
myosin f.
fillet
filter
vena caval f.
filtration
glomerular f.
fimbria, pl. **fimbriae**
f. ovarica
fimbrial
f. evacuation
f. failure
f. obstruction
fimbriectomy
fimbriocele
fimbrioplasty
finding
clinical f.
endovaginal f.
histopathological f.
laboratory f.
pathologic f.
sonographic f.
ultrasonic endovaginal f.
fine-needle
f.-n. aspiration
f.-n. aspiration biopsy
first
f. degree prolapse
f. parallel pelvic plane
f. stage of labor
f. trimester
first-trimester infection
fistula, pl. **fistulae, fistulas**
colovaginal f.
enterovaginal f.
gastrointestinal f.
genitourinary f.
intestinal f.
lacteal f.

low vesicovaginal f.
mammary f.
metroperitoneal f.
perineovaginal f.
postradiation f.
rectolabial f.
rectovaginal f.
rectovestibular f.
rectovulvar f.
tracheoesophageal f.
umbilical f.
urachal f.
ureter fistulae
ureterovaginal f.
urethrovaginal f.
urinary f.
urogenital f.
uteroperitoneal f.
vesicouterine f.
vesicovaginal f.
vesicovaginorectal f.
vitelline f.

Fitz-Hugh and Curtis syndrome

five-year survival rate

fixation

complement f.

Flagyl

flank pain

flap

bulbocavernosus fat f.
fat f.
Martius procedure-bulbocavernosus fat f.
myocutaneous f.

flash

hot f.

flat

f. pelvis
f. wart

flatus vaginalis

flavoxate hydrochloride

flecainide acetate

fleshy mole

Fletcher rule of irradiation tolerance

Fletcher-Suit

F.-S. applicator
F.-S. system for radium therapy

flexion

flood

flooding

floor

pelvic f.

flora

microbial f.

flow

blood f.
cerebral blood f.
cutaneous blood f.
Doppler f.
fetal blood f.
myocardial blood f.
plug f.
pulmonary blood f.
f. rate
renal plasma f.
retrograde menstrual f.
umbilical blood f.
urine f.
uterine blood f.
uteroplacental blood f.
f. velocity waveform
volume f.

Fluanxol

fluconazole

flucytosine

flufenamic acid

fluid

amniotic f.
body f.
cerebrospinal f.
extracellular f.
follicular f.
peritoneal f.
peritoneal cavity f.
f. replacement
f. therapy
transcapillary f.

fluocinolone acetonide

Fluogen

fluorescein-conjugated monoclonal antibody test

fluorescent

f. polarization
f. treponemal antibody absorption (FTA-ABS)

fluorescent-activated cell sorter (FACS)

fluoride

slow-release sodium f.
sodium f.

fluorinated corticosteroid

5-fluorocytosine

fluorodeoxyuridine (FUDR)

9-fluorohydrocortisone
fluorometric immunoassay (FIA)
fluorophosphate
  diisopropyl f.
Fluoroplex
fluorouracil
5-fluorouracil (5-FU)
  intraperitoneal 5-f.
Fluothane
fluoxetine hydrochloride
flupenthixol
fluphenazine
flurazepam
flurbiprofen
flush
  hot f.
  sex f.
flutter
  atrial f.
Fluzone
foam
  intravaginal f.
  f. stability test
focal
  f. change
  f. fibrosis
  f. lobular carcinoma
  f. spot size
focally dilated duct
focus
  endometriotic f.
folate
fold
  Duncan's f.'s
  genitocrural f.
  f. of Hoboken
  rectouterine f.
  urogenital f.
Foldan
folding frequency
Foley catheter
folic
  f. acid
  f. acid antagonist
folinic acid
follicle
  antral f.
  atretic f.
  dominant f.
  graafian f.
  luteinized f.
  luteinized unruptured f.
  f. maturation stimulation
  nabothian f.
  preantral f.
  preovulatory f.
  primary f.
  primordial f.
  f. regulatory protein (FRP)
  f. steroidogenesis
  f. stimulating hormone binding inhibitor
follicle-stimulating
  f.-s. hormone (FSH)
  f.-s. hormone antagonist
  f.-s. hormone inhibition
  f.-s. hormone inhibitor
  f.-s. hormone secretion
follicular
  f. adenocarcinoma of thyroid
  f. attrition
  f. cyst
  f. development arrest
  f. factor
  f. fluid
  f. function
  f. hematoma
  f. maturation
  f. phase
  f. phase gonadotropin secretion
  f. urethritis
  f. vulvitis
folliculogenesis
folliculostatin
follistatin
follow-up
  f.-u. care
  long-term f.-u.
Folvite
fontanel
Food and Drug Administration
foot-drop
footling, foot
  f. presentation
footprinting
foramen ovale
Forane
force
  compression f.
  DES task f.
  expulsive f.
  physician-applied f.
forced expiratory volume

forceps
Adson f.
alligator f.
Allis f.
axis-traction f.
Barton's f.
Baumberger f.
Billroth tumor f.
Bill traction handle f.
Bozeman uterine dressing f.
cephalic f.
Chamberlen f.
Crile f.
DeBakey tissue f.
DeLee f.
f. delivery
DeWees f.
Dewey f.
dressing f.
Elliot f.
Eppendorf punch biopsy f.
failed f.
Haig-Fergusson f.
Halsted mosquito f.
Hawk-Dennen f.
Heaney-Ballentine f.
Heaney-Hyst f.
Hodge's f.
Kevorkian-Younge biopsy f.
Kjelland-Barton f.
Kjelland-Luikart f.
Kjelland's f.
Lahey f.
Laufe polyp f.
Levret's f.
low f.
Luikart f.
f. maneuver
McLean f.
Naegele f.
nonfenestrated f.
obstetrical f.
Ochsner f.
Péan f.
pelvic f.
Phaneuf uterine artery f.
Piper's f.
punch biopsy f.
Randall stone f.
Roch-Ochs f.
Roch-Péan f.
f. rotation
Russian tissue f.
Schroeder tenaculum f.
Schroeder vulsella f.
Schubert uterine biopsy f.
Shute f.
Simpson's f.
Singley f.
sponge f.
sponge holding f.
Tarnier's axis-traction f.
Thomas-Gaylor biopsy f.
tissue f.
trial f.
Tucker-McLean f.
Tucker-McLean-Luikhart f.
Willett's f.
foreign
f. body
f. body salpingitis
foremilk
forewaters
fork
replication f.
form
comedo and cribriform f.
Doppler flow-velocity wave f.
formaldehyde
formation
blood vessel f.
bone f.
chiasma f.
echo f.
somite f.
forme fruste, pl. **formes frustes**
formula
menstrual f.
fornix
Forssman antigen
fosinopril
fossa
f. navicularis
f. ovarica
Fothergill's operation
four-cell embryo
four-chamber view
fourchette
four-hour rule
fourth parallel pelvic plane
Fox-Fordyce disease
fraction
plasma f.
S phase f.
fractional dilation and curettage

fractionation
fracture
birth f.
Colles' f.
fetal f.
hip f.
intrauterine f.
maternal f.
osteoporotic f.
pelvic f.
f. rate
skull f.
spinal compression f.
vertebral compression f.
fragile
f. X carrier
f. X chromosome
f. X syndrome
fragment
Okazaki f.
placental f.
frank
f. breech presentation
Frankenhäuser's plexus
Frankenhüser's ganglion
Franklin-Dukes test
Frank-Starling principle
Frank technique of dilation
free
f. androgen index
f. estradiol
f. fatty acid
f. hydroxyl radical
f. testosterone
f. testosterone index
f. thyroxine index
freezing process
Frei test
French lock
frenectomy
frenoplasty
frenotomy
frequency
folding f.
Nyquist f.
pulse f.
urinary f.
fresh frozen plasma (FFP)
Freund's
F. adjuvant
F. operation
Friberg microsurgical agglutination test
Friedman
F. curve
F. rabbit test
F. test
frontoanterior position
frontoposterior position
frontotransverse position
FRP
follicle regulatory protein
fructose intolerance
frusemide
fruste
forme f.
FSH
follicle-stimulating hormone
FTA-ABS
fluorescent treponemal antibody absorption
5-FU
5-fluorouracil
fucosidosis
FUDR
fluorodeoxyuridine
fulguration
full breech presentation
full-term pregnancy
Fulvicin
function
adrenocortical f.
bladder f.
bowel f.
cardiac f.
cardiorespiratory f.
corpus luteum f.
fetal cardiac f.
fetoplacental f.
follicular f.
hypothalamic-pituitary f.
kidney f.
leukocyte f.
luteal f.
myocardial f.
ovarian f.
pituitary gland f.
pituitary-ovarian f.
pulmonary f.
renal f.
renal tubular f.
reproductive f.
sexual f.
thyroid f.
urethral f.
ventricular f.

functional
f. dysmenorrhea
f. ovarian cyst
f. residual capacity
fundal height
fundectomy
fundus, pl. **fundi**
fundusectomy
fungal infection
Fungizone
fungus, pl. **fungi**
umbilical f.
funic souffle
funicular souffle
funiculus, pl. **funiculi**
f. umbilicalis
funis
funnel-shaped pelvis
Furadantin
Furalan
furan
Furatoin
furazolidone
furosemide
Furoxone
fusanic acid
fusion
labial f.
müllerian duct f.
robertsonian f.
Fusobacterium

G

G
G band
G protein
G_0
gap_0
G_1
gap_1
G_2
gap_2
GAG
glycosaminoglycan
gain
weight g.
galactacrasia
galactagogue
galactic
galactobolic
galactocele
galactography
galactopoiesis
galactopoietic
galactorrhea
galactosemia
galactosis
galactotherapy
galea
gallbladder
g. disease
gallstone
g. pancreatitis
gamete
aging g.
g. intrafallopian transfer (GIFT)
g. manipulation
gametogenesis
ovarian g.
gamma
g. globulin
g. interferon
g. ray
gamma-benzene hexachloride
Gamma BHC
ganglion
Frankenhüser's g.
g. trigger theory
ganglionic blocker
gangliosidosis
generalized g.
juvenile g.
gangrene
spontaneous g. of newborn
Gantanol
Gantrisin
GAP
gonadotropin releasing hormone-associated peptide
gap_0 (G_0)
gap_1 (G_1)
gap_2 (G_2)
gap junction
Garamycin
Gardnerella
G. vaginalis
G. vaginalis chorioamnionitis
gargantuan mastitis
Gariel's pessary
Gartner's
G. cyst
G. duct
gas
g. anesthetic
arterial blood g.
blood g.
g. embolus
fetal blood g.
intervillous blood g.
g. transfer
GASA
growth-adjusted sonographic age
gastric
g. aspiration
g. bypass
g. dysrhythmia
g. emptying time
g. fluid aspiration
g. reduction surgery
Gastrografin
gastrointestinal
g. complication of radiation therapy
g. disorder
g. fistula
g. infection
g. malignancy
g. obstruction
g. series
g. tract
gastroplasty

gastroschisis
gastrostomy
Gaucher's disease
Gauss' sign
GCI
gestational carbohydrate intolerance
G-CSF
granulocyte colony-stimulating factor
GDM
gestational diabetes
gel
prostaglandin E_2 g.
gelastic seizure
gelatin agglutination test
gelatinous varix
Gelpi perineal retractor
gel-transfer
gemellipara
gemmule
Hoboken's g.'s
Gemonil
Genapax
gene
g. action
g. cloning
c-*myc* g.
g. deletion
g. duplication
g. location
g. map
g. mapping
marker g.
g. mutation
od g.
tdy g.
g. therapy
X-linked g.
general anesthesia
generalized gangliosidosis
genesial cycle
genetic
g. abnormality
g. amniocentesis
g. anomaly
g. code
g. counseling
g. diagnosis
g. linkage
g. locus
g. marker
g. material
g. screening
g. susceptibility
genetics
prenatal g.
reproductive g.
genital
g. ambiguity
g. corpuscle
g. development
g. differentiation
g. duct
g. herpes
g. infection
g. lesion
g. mycoplasma
g. ridge
g. tract
g. tract embryology
g. tract malignancy
g. tract trauma
g. tubercle
g. ulcer
g. wart
genitalia
ambiguous g.
external g.
internal g.
lymphatic drainage of g.
genitalis
herpes g.
genitocrural fold
genitourinary
g. abnormality
g. defect
g. fistula
genome
Genora 0.5/35
Genora 1/35
Genora 1/50
genotype
gentamicin
gentian violet
genucubital position
genupectoral position
Geocillin
Geopen
geophagia
Gepfert procedure
geriatrics
germ
g. cell
g. cell ovarian neoplasm
g. cell ovarian tumor

g. cell tumor
g. layer
German
G. lock
G. measles
germinal
g. epithelium
g. epithelium of Waldeyer
g. vesicle
gestagen
gestagenic
gestation
anembryonic g.
multiple g.
prolonged g.
term g.
tubal g.
twin g.
unruptured tubal g.
gestational
g. abnormality
g. age
g. age estimation
g. carbohydrate intolerance (GCI)
g. diabetes (GDM)
g. edema
g. hypertension
g. proteinuria
g. psychosis
g. ring
g. sac mean diameter
g. sac observation
g. trophoblastic disease (GTD)
g. trophoblastic neoplasia (GTN)
g. trophoblastic tumor
Gestogen
gestosis, pl. **gestoses**
Gestrinone
GF
growth factor
GFR
glomerular filtration rate
GH
growth hormone
GH-RH
growth hormone-releasing hormone
giant
g. baby
g. fibroadenoma
Gianturco spring
Giemsa stain
GIFT
gamete intrafallopian transfer
cervical GIFT
intrauterine GIFT
vaginal GIFT
gigantomastia
Gigli's
G. operation
G. saw
Gilliam's operation
gingivitis
gitalin
gland
adrenal g.
apocrine g.
Bartholin's g.
bulbourethral g.
eccrine g.
endocrine g.
fetal adrenal g.
mammary g.
Montgomery's g.'s
parathyroid g.
paraurethral g.
periurethral g.
pineal g.
pituitary g.
salivary g.
Skene's g.
thymus g.
thyroid g.
urethral g.
uterine g.
vestibular g.
glandular
g. hyperplasia
g. mastitis
g. tissue
glans
glassy cell carcinoma
Glaucon
gleet
gleety
gliosis
g. uteri
globin
α-globin
β-globin
globulin
anti-D gamma g.
anti-D immune g.

globulin *(continued)*
antithymocyte g.
corticosteroid-binding g. (CBG)
gamma g.
hepatitis B immune g.
hepatitis immune g.
immune g.
immune serum g. (ISG)
pregnancy-associated g.
rabies immune g.
RH_o (D) immune g.
sex hormone-binding g. (SHBG)
testosterone-estrogen-binding g.
tetanus immune g.
thyroid-binding g. (TBG)
thyroxine-binding g.
varicella-zoster immune g.
zoster immune g.
glomerular
g. capillary endotheliosis
g. change
g. filtration
g. filtration rate (GFR)
glomerulonephritis
membranous g.
glomerulopathy
glomerulosclerosis
gloving
double g.
glucagon
glucocorticoid
glucocorticosteroid therapy
gluconate
potassium g.
glucose
blood g.
g. challenge test
fetal blood g.
hypertonic g.
g. intolerance
g. meter
g. tolerance
urinary g.
glucose-6-phosphate dehydrogenase
glucosiduronate
glucosuria
glucuronate pregnanediol
glucuronide
3α-androstanediol g.
5α-androstane-3α,17β-diol g. (3α-diol-G)
androsterone g.
virilizing 3α-androstanediol g.
gluteal node
glycemic control
glycerin
glycerol
iodinated g.
glycerophospholipid
glyceryl guaiacolate
glycogen-storage disease
glycoprotein
glycopyrrolate
glycosaminoglycan (GAG)
glycoside
cardiac g.
glycosuria
glycosylated hemoglobin A
Glyrol
GM-CSF
granulocyte-macrophage colony-stimulating factor
GnRH
gonadotropin-releasing hormone
GnRH-facilitated
G.-f. FSH release
G.-f. LH release
Goebell-Stoeckel-Frangenheim procedure
GOG
Gynecologic Oncology Group
goiter
simple colloid g.
gold
radioactive g.
g. salt
g. sodium thiomalate
gold-198 (^{198}Au)
GoLYTELY
gonad
maternal g.
undifferentiated g.
gonadal
g. agenesis
g. axis
g. dysgenesis
g. failure
g. ridge
g. sex
g. steroid suppression
g. streak

g. stroma
g. stromal ovarian tumor
gonadectomy
gonadoblastoma
ovarian g.
gonadocrinin
gonadostat
gonadotrope
gonadotrophin-releasing hormone-like protein
gonadotrophin-resistant ovary syndrome
gonadotropin, gonadotrophin
chorionic g. (CG)
exogenous g.
human chorionic g. (HCG, hCG)
human menopausal g. (HMG)
pituitary g.
pulsatile human menopausal g.
g. pulsatile release
g. regulation
g. release
g. releasing hormone-associated peptide (GAP)
g. secretion
g. secretion inhibitor
gonadotropin-induced ovarian hyperstimulation
gonadotropin-releasing
g.-r. hormone (GnRH)
g.-r. hormone agonist
g.-r. hormone analogue
g.-r. hormone antagonist
g.-r. hormone-like peptide
g.-r. peptide
gonadotropin-resistant testis
gonane
gonoblennorrhea
gonococcal
g. conjunctivitis
g. infection
gonococcus
gonorrhea
disseminated g.
gonorrheal
g. cervicitis
g. ophthalmia
g. salpingitis
gonozyme test
Goodall-Power modification
Goodell's
G. dilator
G. sign
gossypol
Goulet retractor
Gower-1
hemoglobin G.
Gower-2
hemoglobin G.
Gower's sign
graafian follicle
gracilis muscle
grade
placental g.
grading
histopathological g.
placental g.
Graefenberg ring
graft
allogeneic fetal g.
bilateral myocutaneous g.
heterologous g.
isogeneic g.
split-thickness g.
graft-versus-host reaction
Gram-negative organism
Gram-positive
G.-p. cocci
G.-p. rod
Gram's stain
grand
g. climacteric
g. multifetal pregnancy
g. multipara
g. multiparity
grandmother theory
granular
g. cell myoblastoma
g. urethritis
granulation tissue
granule
cortical g.
Langerhans' g.
sulfur g.
granulocyte colony-stimulating factor (G-CSF)
granulocyte-macrophage colony-stimulating factor (GM-CSF)
granuloma
g. gravidarum
g. inguinale
Langhans' giant cell g.
pyogenic g.

granulomatosis
Wegener's g.
granulomatous
g. calcification
g. infection
g. mastitis
g. salpingitis
granulosa
g. cell
g. lutein cell
granulosa-stromal cell tumor
granulosa-theca cell tumor
grape mole
Graves
G. bivalve speculum
G. disease
G. speculum
gravid
g. uterus
gravida
gravida I
gravida II
gravidarum
chorea g.
hyperemesis g.
gravidic
g. retinitis
g. retinopathy
gravidism
graviditas
g. examnialis
g. exochorialis
gravidity
gravis
icterus g.
myasthenia g.
Gravol
gray
g. baby syndrome
g. syndrome
gray-scale ultrasonography
great vessel
Green uterine curette
grid
Grifulvin V
Grisactin
griseofulvin
Grisovin
Gris-PEG
groin
g. dissection
g. hernia
groove
neural g.
primitive g.
g. sign
group
g. A beta-hemolytic streptococcus
blood g.
g. B streptococcus
determinant g.
g. D streptococcus
Rh blood g.
support g.
growth
bacterial g.
g. discordancy
g. factor (GF)
fetal g.
fetal cellular g.
g. hormone (GH)
g. hormone-releasing hormone (GH-RH)
g. hormone-secreting adenoma
longitudinal g.
non-estrogen-regulated g.
placental g.
g. problem
pubertal g.
g. retardation
retarded fetal g.
skeletal g.
growth-adjusted sonographic age (GASA)
growth-discordant twin
growth-like factor
growth-retarded fetus
G-spot
GTD
gestational trophoblastic disease
GTN
gestational trophoblastic neoplasia
GTP
guanosine 5′-triphosphate
guaiacolate
glyceryl g.
guaiac test
guaifenesin
guanabenz
guanadrel
guanethidine
guanfacine

guanine
guanosine 5′-triphosphate (GTP)
gubernaculum
guidance
ultrasound g.
Guillain-Barré syndrome
gumma
gut suture
GYN
gynecologic
gynecologist
gynecology
gynandroblastoma
gynatresia
gynecic
gynecogenic
gynecography
gynecoid
g. obesity
g. pelvis
gynecologic, gynecological (GYN)
g. cancer
g. history
Gynecologic Oncology Group (GOG)
gynecologist (GYN)
Gynecologists
American College of Obstetricians and G.
gynecology (GYN)
adolescent g.
pediatric g.
gynecomastia
Gyne-Lotrimin
gyniatrics
gyniatry
Gynogen L.A.
Gynol II
gynopathy
gynoplasty, gynoplastics

H

Haase's rule
habit
bowel h.'s
eating h.'s
sex h.'s
habitual abortion
habitus
fetal h.
HAC
hexamethylmelamine with doxorubicin and cyclophosphamide
Haemophilus
H. ducreyi
Haig-Fergusson forceps
hair
h. growth phase
h. loss
pubic h.
sexual h.
terminal h.
vellus h.
HAIR-AN
hyperandrogenism, insulin resistance, acanthosis nigricans
hairpin vessel
Halban's syndrome
Haldol
half-life
half-value layer (HVL)
halo
fatty h.
h. sign
haloperidol
halothane
Halsted
H. mosquito forceps
Halstedian concept of tumor spread
Halsted's operation
hamartoma
hamster
h. egg penetration assay
h. ovum
hand
h. abnormality
h. bone abnormality
Hanks
H. uterine dilator
Hansen's disease
H_2-antagonist
histamine H.-a.
haplotype
maternal HLA h.
hapten
harlequin
h. fetus
h. reaction
Harrington retractor
Hartman's sign
Hartnup disease
Hashimoto's thyroiditis
hashish
Hashitoxicosis
HATTS
hemagglutination treponemal test
Hawk-Dennen forceps
HBsAg
hepatitis B surface antigen
HCG, hCG
human chorionic gonadotropin
β-HCG
human chorionic gonadotropin beta-subunit
HDL
high-density lipoprotein
HDL-cholesterol
head
breech h.
h. circumference/abdominal circumference ratio
h. compression
dolichocephalic h.
fetal h.
hourglass h.
h. presentation
headache
migraine h.
preeclampsia h.
spinal h.
vascular h.
head:body ratio
health
fetal h.
Health Insurance Plan (HIP)
Heaney
H. clamp
H. curette

Heaney *(continued)*
H. needle holder
H. operation
Heaney-Ballentine forceps
Heaney-Hyst
H.-H. forceps
H.-H. retractor
heart
h. block
h. disease
h. failure
fetal h.
h. rate
h. rate monitoring
h. sound
h. valve replacement
heartburn
heart-shaped
h.-s. pelvis
h.-s. uterus
heat
h. loss
h. transfer mechanism
Hegar's
H. dilators
H. sign
height
fundal h.
h. table
helcomenia
helix
double h.
HELLP syndrome
Helmex
helper
h. factor
h. T cell
hemagglutinating inhibition antibody (HIA)
hemagglutination inhibition
hemagglutination treponemal test (HATTS)
hemagglutinin
hemagogue
hemangioma
epidural h.
vulvar h.
hematocele
pelvic h.
pudendal h.
hematocolpometra
hematocolpos
hematocrit
mean menstrual cycle h.
hematologic
h. disorder
h. neoplasia
hematology
hematoma
axillary h.
h. drainage
follicular h.
interstitial and loculated h.
intrauterine h.
puerperal h.
uterine h.
vaginal h.
vulvar h.
hematometra
hematomphalocele
hematopoiesis
extramedullary h.
hematopoietic
h. system
hematosalpinx
hematotrachelos
hematuria
hemelytrometra
heme metabolism disorder
hemicervix
hemiuterus
hemivulvectomy
hemochorial placenta
hemochorioendothelial placentation
hemoconcentration
hemodialysis
hemodynamic monitoring
hemodynamics
hemoglobin
h. A
h. A_{Ic}
h. Bart's
h. C
h. E
h. F
fetal h.
h. Gower-1
h. Gower-2
h. H
h. Portland
h. S
hemoglobinemia
hemoglobinopathy
hemoglobinuria
paroxysmal nocturnal h.

hemolysin
hemolysis
microangiopathic h.
hemolytic
ABO h. disease of the newborn
h. anemia
h. disease of the newborn
h. uremic syndrome
β-hemolytic streptococcus
hemometra
hemoperitoneum
hemophilia
h. A
h. B
hemoptysis
hemorrhage
accidental h.
antepartum h.
concealed h.
external h.
fetal h.
fetal-maternal h.
fetal-to-maternal h.
intracranial h.
intrapartum h.
intraventricular h.
placental h.
postpartum h.
subarachnoid h.
subchorionic h.
transplacental h.
unavoidable h.
hemorrhagic
h. cystitis
h. endovasculitis
h. shock
hemorrhoid
hemorrhoidal
h. artery
h. nerve
hemosalpinx
hemostasis
hemostat
Crile h.
curved h.
Henderson-Hasselbalch equation
Hepalean
heparin
calcium h.
h. challenge test
low-dose h.
minidose h.
prophylactic h.
h. sodium
hepatic
h. focal nodular hyperplasia
h. metastasis
h. necrosis
h. neoplasm
h. pregnancy
h. rupture
hepatitis
h. A
h. A virus
h. B
h. B immune globulin
h. B surface antigen (HBsAg)
h. B vaccine
h. B virus
chronic h.
h. D
delta h.
h. immune globulin
h. immunization
infectious h.
maternal h.
non-A, non-B h.
serum h.
hepatocellular
h. carcinoma
h. damage
hepatolenticular degeneration
hepatosplenomegaly
Hep-B-Gammagee
herbicide
Herbst registry
hereditary
h. nonspherocytic anemia
h. orotic aciduria
h. spherocytosis
h. syphilis
heredity
heritability
hermaphrodite
hermaphroditism
true h.
XX h.
HER-2/neu proto-oncogene
hernia
abdominal h.
h. of the broad ligament of the uterus
diaphragmatic h.
epigastric h.

hernia *(continued)*
femoral h.
groin h.
hiatal h.
incarcerated h.
incisional h.
inguinal h.
labial h.
reducible h.
sliding h.
spigelian h.
strangulated h.
umbilical h.
h. uterine inguinale
ventral h.
herpes
genital h.
h. genitalis
h. gestationis
intrauterine h.
h. labialis
neonatal h.
h. simplex
h. simplex virus (HSV)
h. zoster
herpesvirus
h. type 1 (HSV-1)
h. type 2 (HSV-2)
Herplex Liquifilm
Hesselbach's triangle
hetacillin
heterograft
heterologous
h. graft
h. insemination
h. uterine sarcoma
heterophil
h. antigen
heterosexual precocious puberty
heterotopic
h. pregnancy
heterozygosity
heterozygous
h. carrier
Heuser's membrane
Hexa-Betalin
Hexa-CAF
hexamethylmelamine, cyclophosphamide, doxorubicin, and 5-fluorouracil
hexachloride
gamma-benzene h.
hexachlorocyclohexane
Hexadrol
hexamethonium chloride
hexamethylmelamine
hexamethylmelamine, cyclophosphamide, doxorubicin, and 5-fluorouracil (Hexa-CAF)
hexamethylmelamine with doxorubicin and cyclophosphamide (HAC)
hexamine
hexestrol
hexocyclium methylsulfate
hexosaminidase
Heyman's capsules
Heyns' abdominal decompression apparatus
HG factor
HIA
hemagglutinating inhibition antibody
5-HIAA
5-hydroxyindoleacetic acid
hiatal hernia
hiccup
hidradenitis suppurativa
hidradenoma
papillary h.
high
h. altitude perinatal mortality
h. fetal order
h. forceps
h. intrauterine insemination
runner's h.
high-density lipoprotein (HDL)
high-dose chemotherapy
high-fiber diet
high-grade cervical dysplasia
high molecular weight dextran
high-risk
h.-r. mother
h.-r. patient
h.-r. pregnancy
h.-r. pregnancy unit
high-tech obstetrician
hilar cell tumor
Hillis-Müller maneuver
hilus, pl. **hili**
hindwater
HIP
Health Insurance Plan

hip
h. bone density
h. deformity
h. dislocation
h. fracture
Hiprex
Hip-Rex
hirsute
hirsutism
constitutional h.
familial h.
hormonal h.
idiopathic h.
postmenopausal h.
His' rule
histaminase
histamine
h. H_2-antagonist
Histantil
Histatan
histidinuria
histocompatibility
h. antigen
h. locus antigen
histoimmunological origin
histoincompatibility
maternal-fetal h.
histologic architecture
histologic diagnosis
histology
endometrial h.
histone
histopathological
h. diagnosis
h. finding
h. grading
h. study
histopathology
histoplasmosis
historical assessment
history
family h.
gynecologic h.
medical h.
menstrual h.
obstetric h.
occupational h.
reproductive h.
sexual h.
social h.
h. taking
urologic h.
HIV
human immunodeficiency virus
HIV testing
HLA
human leukocyte antigen
HLA-B14,DR1
HLA-compatible fetus
HLI
human leukocyte interferon
HMG
human menopausal gonadotropin
hobnail cells
Hoboken
fold of H.
H. gemmules
H. nodules
Hodge's
H. forceps
H. pessary
Hodgkin's disease
Hofbauer cell
holder
Crile-Wood needle h.
Heaney needle h.
Mayo-Hegar needle h.
Wagenstein needle h.
holoprosencephaly
h. anomalad
Holt-Oram syndrome
Homans' sign
homatropine
home
h. birth
h. pregnancy testing
homocystinuria
homograft
homologous
h. disease
h. insemination
h. uterine sarcoma
homozygous
hood
vaginal h.
horizontal transmission
hormonal
h. antineoplastic therapy
h. contraception
h. effect
h. hirsutism
h. implant
h. pregnancy test tablets

hormone
h. abnormality
adrenocortical h.
adrenocorticotropic h. (ACTH)
anterior pituitary-like h.
antidiuretic h.
h. assay
bioactive h.
calcitropic h.
cancer and steroid h. (CASH)
chorionic gonadotropic h., chorionic gonadotrophic h.
chorionic growth h.
circulating h.
h. complex receptor
corticotropin-releasing h. (CRH)
endogenous h.
exogenous h.
fetal h.
follicle-stimulating h. (FSH)
gonadotropin-releasing h. (GnRH)
growth h. (GH)
growth h.-releasing hormone (GH-RH)
human chorionic adrenocorticotropic h.
luteinizing h. (LH)
luteinizing hormone-releasing h. (LH-RH)
melanocyte-stimulating h.
ovarian h.
parathyroid h.
pituitary h.
placental h.
pregnancy h.
purified h.
h. receptor
recombinant human growth h.
h. replacement therapy
sex h.
steroid h.
h. therapy
thyroid h.
thyroid-stimulating h. (TSH)
thyrotropic h.
thyrotropin-releasing h. (TRH)
tropic h.

hormone-receptor complex internalization

hormone-stimulated endometrial change

horn
noncommunicating uterine h.
rudimentary uterine h.
uterine h., h. of uterus

horseshoe
h. fibrosis
h. placenta

hospice

hospital
h. birth
h. discharge

hospitalization

host
h. defense mechanism
h. response mechanism

hot
h. flash
h. flush

Hottentot apron

hourglass head

24-hour urinary free cortisol

HPL
human placental lactogen

HPV
human papilloma virus

H-ras p21 protein

HSG
hysterosalpingography

HSV
herpes simplex virus

HSV-1
herpesvirus type 1

HSV-2
herpesvirus type 2

HSV-1 encephalitis

HSV-2 encephalitis

HTLV
human T-cell leukemia virus

HTLV-III
human T-cell leukemia virus type III

Huhner test

human
h. chorionic adrenocorticotropic hormone
h. chorionic gonadotropin (HCG, hCG)

h. chorionic gonadotropin beta-subunit (β-HCG)
h. chorionic thyrotropin
h. immunodeficiency virus (HIV)
h. leukocyte antigen (HLA)
h. leukocyte interferon (HLI)
h. lymphocyte antigen
h. menopausal gonadotropin (HMG)
h. ovum fertilization test
h. papilloma virus (HPV)
h. placental lactogen (HPL)
h. T-cell leukemia virus (HTLV)
h. T-cell leukemia virus type III (HTLV-III)

Humatin
humoral
h. antibody
h. factor
h. immunity
Humorsol
Hunter's syndrome
Huntington's disease
Hurler's syndrome
husband
artificial insemination by h. (AIH)
h. washed spermatozoa
Hutterite
HVL
half-value layer
hyaline
h. membrane disease of the newborn
h. myoma degeneration
H-Y antigen
hybridization
DNA h.
Papillomavirus h.
hybridoma technique
Hycodan
hydantoin syndrome
hydatid
h. cyst of Morgagni
h. mole
h. pregnancy
hydatidiform mole
hydralazine hydrochloride
hydramnion, hydramnios
hydranencephaly
Hydrate
hydrate
chloral h.
hydration
maternal h.
Hydra-zide
Hydrea
hydriodic acid
hydroa
h. gestationis
hydrocele
h. feminae
h. muliebris
Nuck's h.
hydrocephalus
hydrocephaly
Hydro-chlor
hydrochloride
hydrochlorothiazide
hydrocodone
hydrocolpocele, hydrocolpos
hydrocortisone
HydroDIURIL
hydroflumethiazide
hydrogen peroxide
hydrometra
hydrometrocolpos
hydromorphone
Hydromox
hydronephrosis
hydroparasalpinx
hydrops
fetal h., h. fetalis
h. folliculi
immune fetal h.
maternal h.
nonimmune fetal h.
h. ovarii
severe fetal h.
h. tubae
h. tubae profluens
hydrorrhea
h. gravidae, h. gravidarum
hydrosalpinx
intermittent h.
hydrothorax
hydrotubation
hydroureter
hydrovarium

hydroxide
magnesium h.
potassium h.
11β-hydroxyandrosterone
17-hydroxycorticosteroid
11-hydroxyetiocholanolone
5-hydroxyindoleacetic acid (5-HIAA)
hydroxyindole-*o*-methyltransferase
hydroxylase
phenylalanine h.
11β-hydroxylase
17-hydroxylase
17α-hydroxylase
21-hydroxylase
21-h. gene
21-h. gene deletion
hydroxylation
3-hydroxy-3-methylglutaryl coenzyme A
hydroxyphenyluria
17-hydroxypregnenolone
17α-hydroxypregnenolone
hydroxyprogesterone
h. caproate
17-hydroxyprogesterone (17-OHP)
17-h. caproate
17α-hydroxyprogesterone
17α-h. caproate
hydroxyprogesterone and estradiol valerate
15-hydroxyprostaglandin dehydrogenase
3β-hydroxysteroid
3β-h. dehydrogenase
18-hydroxysteroid dehydrogenase deficiency
hydroxyurea
25-hydroxyvitamin-D_3
hydroxyzine
hygiene
perineal h.
hygroma
cystic h.
Hygroton
Hylorel
hymen
h. bifenestratus, h. biforis
cribriform h.
denticulate h.
imperforate h.
infundibuliform h.
redundant h.
h. sculptatus
septate h.
h. subseptus
vertical h.
hymenectomy
hymenitis
hymenorrhaphy
hymenotomy
hyoscine
h. methylbromide
hypamnion, hypamnios
Hypaque
Hyperab
hyperalimentation
hyperammonemia
hyperandrogenemia
hyperandrogenism
adrenal h.
cryptic h.
ovarian h.
h. reversal
hyperandrogenism, insulin resistance, acanthosis nigricans (HAIR-AN)
hyperbaric oxygen
hyperbilirubinemia
hypercalcemia
hypercalcemic crisis
hypercalciuria
hypercapnia
hypercarbia
hypercholesterolemia
familial h.
hypercoagulability
hypercortisolism
hypercyesis, hypercyesia
hyperdynamia
h. uteri
hyperemesis
h. gravidarum
h. lactentium
hyperfolliculoidism
hypergalactosis
hyperglycemia
ketotic h.
nonketotic h.
hyperglycinemia
hypergonadotropic, hypergonadotrophic
h. amenorrhea
h. hypogonadism
hypergynecosmia
HyperHep

hyperinsulinemia
hyperinvolution
hyperlactation
hyperlaxity
joint h.
hyperlipidemia
hyperlysinemia
hypermagnesemia
hypermastia
hypermenorrhea
hyperornithinemia
hyperosmotic agent
hyperovarianism
hyperoxia
hyperparathyroidism
maternal h.
hyperphenylalaninemia
hyperpigmentation
hyperpigmented lesion
hyperplasia
adenomatous h.
adenomatous endometrial h.
adrenal h.
adult-onset congenital adrenal h.
congenital h.
congenital adrenal h.
cystic h.
cystic h. of the breast
cystic glandular h.
ductal h.
endometrial h. (EH)
epithelial h.
familial lipoid adrenal h.
fetal congenital h.
glandular h.
hepatic focal nodular h.
hilar cell h.
late-onset h.
lipoid adrenal h.
microglandular cervical h.
polypoid h.
Swiss cheese h.
vulvar squamous h.
hyperprolactinemia
tumorous h.
hyperprolactinemia-associated luteal phase
hyperprolactinemic amenorrhea
hyperreactio luteinalis
hyperreflexia
hyperrelaxinemia
hypersecretion
hypersensitivity
delayed h.
Hyperstat
hyperstimulation
gonadotropin-induced ovarian h.
ovarian h.
hypertension
chronic h.
gestational h.
intracranial h.
maternal h.
portal h.
postpartum h.
pregnancy-induced h.
pulmonary h.
hypertensive
h. drug
h. encephalopathy
Hyper-Tet
hyperthecosis
stromal h.
hyperthermia
hyperthyroidism
hypertonic
h. glucose
h. saline
h. uterine dysfunction
hypertrichosis
hypertrophic cirrhosis
hypertrophy
massive breast h.
myocardial h.
virginal breast h.
hypervalinemia
hyperventilation
hyperviscosity
h. syndrome
hypnotic effect
hypoadrenalism
hypocalcemia
neonatal h.
hypocycloidal tomography
hypoestrogenic
h. rate
h. woman
hypofertility
hypofibrinogenemia
congenital h.
familial h.
hypofolliculogenesis
hypogalactia
hypogalactous

hypogastric
h. artery
h. lymph node
h. pain
h. plexus
hypoglycemia
neonatal h.
hypoglycemic
oral h.
hypogonadal
hypogonadism
eugonadotropic h.
hypergonadotropic h.
hypogonadotropic h.
hypogonadotropic
h. amenorrhea
h. hypogonadism
hypokalemia
hypomagnesemia
hypomastia, hypomazia
hypomenorrhea
hypoovarianism, hypovarianism
hypoparathyroidism
hypophosphatasia
hypophyseal portal circulation
hypophysectomy
hypophysial, hypophyseal
hypophysial amenorrhea
hypophysitis
lymphocytic h.
hypopituitarism
hypoplasia
congenital adrenal h.
lipoid adrenal gland h.
müllerian h.
pulmonary h.
hypoplastic
h. anemia
h. lung
h. penis
hypospadias
hypotension
maternal h.
orthostatic h.
hypothalamic
h. amenorrhea
h. disease
h. dysfunction
h. failure
hypothalamic-hypophyseal-ovarian-endometrial axis
hypothalamic-hypophyseal portal circulation
hypothalamic-pituitary
h.-p. axis
h.-p. disorder
h.-p. dysfunction
h.-p. function
hypothalamic-pituitary-gonadal axis
hypothalamus
hypothermia
chronic scrotal h.
hypothesis
critical weight h.
estrogen window etiologic h.
Korenman's estrogen window h.
Lyon h.
null h.
hypothyroidism
congenital h.
subclinical h.
transient congenital h.
hypotonic
h. myometrium
h. uterine dysfunction
hypovolemia
hypovolemic shock
hypoxia
fetal h.
hypoxic
h. cell sensitizer
h. ischemic encephalopathy
Hyproval
Hyrexin
Hyskon
hysteralgia
hysteratresia
hysterectomy
abdominal h.
abdominovaginal h.
cesarean h.
extrafascial h.
Meigs-Werthein h.
modified radical h.
obstetrical h.
paravaginal h.
Porro h.
radical h.
Rutledge classification of extended h.
subtotal h.
supracervical h.
total abdominal h. (TAH)
vaginal h.
hystereurysis

hysterocele
hysterocleisis
hysterocolposcope
hysterocystopexy
hysterodynia
hysterogram
hysterograph
hysterography
hysterolith
hysterolysis
hysterometer
hysteromyoma
hysteromyomectomy
hysteromyotomy
hystero-oophorectomy
hysteropathy
hysteropexy
abdominal h.
hysterophore
hysteroplasty
hysterorrhaphy
hysterorrhexis
hysterosalpingectomy
hysterosalpingography (HSG)
hysterosalpingo-oophorectomy
hysterosalpingostomy
hysteroscope
hysteroscopic
h. removal
h. surgery
hysteroscopy
hysterospasm
hysterothermometry
hysterotomy
abdominal h.
vaginal h.
hysterotonin
hysterotrachelectomy
hysterotracheloplasty
hysterotrachelorrhaphy
hysterotrachelotomy
hysterotubography
Hytakerol
Hytuss

I

^{125}I
iodine-125
^{131}I
iodine-131
iatrogenic
i. dissemination
i. event
i. fetal distress
i. menopause
i. precocious puberty
i. ureteral injury
ibuprofen
I-cell disease
ichthyosis
i. uteri
ICRF 159
icterus
i. gravis
i. neonatorum
physiologic i.
IDDM
insulin-dependent diabetes mellitus
idiopathic
i. cholestasis of pregnancy
i. hirsutism
i. hypertrophic subaortic stenosis
i. infertility
i. precocious puberty
i. thrombocytopenic purpura (ITP)
idoxuridine
IFN
interferon
ifosfamide
Ig
immunoglobulin
IgA
immunoglobulin A
secretory IgA
IGF
insulin-like growth factor
IgG
immunoglobulin G
IgM
immunoglobulin M
IgM antibody
IL
interleukin
IL-1
interleukin-1
IL-2
interleukin-2
ileal
i. conduit
i. perforation
ileocolic artery
ileoentectropy
ileostomy
continent i.
ileus
adynamic i.
meconium i.
paralytic i.
i. subparta
iliac
i. artery
i. node
i. vein
iliococcygeal muscle
iliofemoral thrombosis
ilioneoureterocystotomy
iliopectineal line
ill-defined mass
illicit drug use
illness
psychiatric i.
systemic i.
Ilosone
Ilotycin
image recording system
imaging
diagnostic i.
fetal i.
magnetic resonance i. (MRI)
radiologist-referred diagnostic i.
Rh_o (D) i.
self-referred diagnostic i.
imbalance
electrolyte i.
imidazole
iminoglycinuria
imipramine hydrochloride
Imlach's ring
immature ovarian teratoma
imminent abortion

immobilization
Treponema pallidum i. (TPI)
immune
i. clearance
i. factor
i. fetal hydrops
i. globulin
i. monitoring technique
i. process
i. rejection
i. response
i. separation technique
i. serum globulin (ISG)
i. state
i. surveillance
i. system
i. thrombocytopenia
i. thrombocytopenic purpura (ITP)
immunity
cell-mediated i. (CMI)
cellular i.
humoral i.
passive i.
previous maternal i.
immunization
blood group i.
hepatitis i.
prophylactic i.
Rh i.
immunoassay
chemiluminescent i. (CIA)
enzyme i.
fluorometric i. (FIA)
nonradioactive i.
nonreactive i.
radioactive i.
solid-phase enzyme i.
Immunobead test
immunochemistry
immunochemotherapy
immunocompetent cell
immunodeficiency
combined i.
i. syndrome
immunodiagnosis
immunofluorescence
immunofluorescent antibody test
immunogen
immunogenetics
immunoglobulin (Ig)
i. A (IgA)
i. administration
antenatal anti-D i.
anti-D i.
i. G (IgG)
intravenous i.
intravenous anti-D i.
i. M (IgM)
Rh i.
$Rh_o(D)$ i.
surface i.
thyroid-stimulating i.
immunohistochemical
i. change
i. stromal leukocyte characterization
immunologic, immunological
i. assay
i. change
i. enhancement
i. paralysis
i. pregnancy test
i. rejection
i. suppression
i. surveillance
i. tolerance
i. unresponsiveness
immunology
maternal i.
placental i.
transplantation i.
tumor i.
immunoprophylaxis
immunoprotein
immunoradiometric assay (IRMA)
immunoreaction
immunoreactivity
immunoresistance
immunosuppression
immunosuppressive
i. therapy
immunotherapy
adoptive i.
nonspecific i.
specific i.
systemic-active nonspecific i.
tumor i.
Imodium
Imogam
Imovax
impacted fetus
impaction
fecal i.
impaired secretion

impairment
inherited androgen uptake i.
opioidergic control i.
impedance plethysmography
imperforate
i. anus
i. hymen
impetigo
i. herpetiformis
implant
collapsed subpectoral i.
endometrial i.
hormonal i.
peritoneal i.
saline i.
silicone i.
subdermal i.
subpectoral i.
transperineal i.
transvaginal i.
implantation
cortical i.
i. failure
i. phase
placental i.
i. theory of the production of endometriosis
tubouterine i.
Impril
Imuran
^{111}In
indium-111
in
inactivated poliovirus vaccine
inactivation pattern
inactive endometrium
inadequacy
luteal phase i.
inadequate
i. luteal phase
i. surgery
inappropriate lactation
Inapsine
inborn errors of metabolism
incarcerated
i. hernia
i. placenta
incessant ovulation
incest
incipient abortion
incision
abdominal i.
cervical i.
classical transverse i.
i. closure
colpotomy i.
Kehr i.
laparotomy i.
low-segment transverse i.
Maylard i.
midline i.
paramedian i.
Pfannenstiel's i.
Sanger i.
Sellheim i.
superumbilical i.
supraumbilical i.
uterine i.
incisional hernia
inclination
pelvic i.
inclusion cyst
incompatibility
ABO i.
incompatible blood group antigen
incompetence
cervical i. (CI)
incompetent
i. cervix
incomplete
i. abortion
i. foot presentation
i. knee presentation
i. precocious puberty
i. puberty
i. testicular feminization
incontinence
anal i.
i. of milk
overflow i.
paradoxical i.
true i.
urge i.
urinary i.
urinary exertional i.
urinary stress i.
increase
plasma prorenin i.
short-term i.
incubation
incubator
incudiform uterus
indapamide
Inderal
index, gen. **indicis**, pl. **indices, indexes**

index *(continued)*
body mass i.
i. case
deoxyribonucleic acid i.
free androgen i.
free testosterone i.
free thyroxine i.
karyopyknotic i.
Pearl i.
pelvic i.
ponderal i.
Pourcelot i.
pulsatility i.
resistance i.
Stuart i.
testosterone i.
thyroid i.
total testosterone i.
urinary diagnostic i. (UDI)
indicator
prognostic i.
indifferent gonadal stage
indigenous neoplasm
indigo carmine
indigotin
indirect
i. maternal death
i. ovular transmigration
i. placentography
indium-111 (^{111}In)
Indocid
Indocin
indolamine
indomethacin
induced
i. abortion
i. labor
i. remission
induction
labor augmentation i.
menstrual cycle i.
ovulation i.
superovulation i.
indusium, pl. **indusia**
inefficiency
female fertility i.
inertia
uterine i., primary
uterine i., secondary
uterine i., true uterine i.
inevitable abortion
infant
i. death
i. of diabetic mother
drug-depressed i.
large-for-date i.
liveborn i.
low-birth-weight i.
i. morbidity
i. mortality
i. mortality rate
postterm i.
premature i.
preterm i.
Rh-positive i.
small-for-gestational-age i.
stillborn i.
term i.
very-low-birth-weight i.
infantile
i. spasm
i. spastic paraplegia
infarct
placental i.
uric acid i.
white i.
infarction
cerebral i.
myocardial i.
pulmonary i.
infected abortion
infection
adnexal i.
amniotic cavity bacterial i.
asymptomatic i.
bacterial i.
benign *Papillomavirus* i.
cervical i.
cervicovaginal i.
chlamydial i.
chorioamnionic i.
cytomegalovirus i.
disseminated i.
fetal i.
first-trimester i.
fungal i.
gastrointestinal i.
genital i.
gonococcal i.
granulomatous i.
intra-amniotic i.
intrauterine i.
IUD-related i.
latent herpes simplex virus i.
lower genital tract i.

maternal i.
neisserial i.
neonatal i.
nosocomial i.
Papillomavirus i.
pelvic i.
pharyngeal gonococcal i.
postpartum i.
puerperal i.
recurrent i.
respiratory i.
respiratory tract i.
retroperitoneal i.
streptococcal i.
surgical i.
symptomatic i.
Trichomonas i.
upper genital tract i.
urinary tract i.
uterine i.
vaginal i.
varicella i.
varicella-zoster virus i.
vertically acquired i.
viral i.
vulvar i.
vulvovaginal premenarchal i.
wound i.
yeast i.
infectious hepatitis
infective endocarditis
infecundity
inferior
inferior i.
i. mesenteric artery
i. vena cava
infertile
infertility
i. agent
anovulatory i.
asymptomatic i.
endometriosis-associated i.
i. evaluation
i. factor
familial i.
idiopathic i.
inherited i.
i. investigation
male i.
male factor i.
primary i.
secondary i.
unexplained i.
infiltrating
i. carcinoma
i. ductal carcinoma
i. lobular carcinoma
i. small cell lobular carcinoma
infiltration
fatty i.
inflammation
pelvic i.
inflammatory
i. bowel disease
i. carcinoma
influenza
i. A
i. vaccine
i. virus
informed
i. consent
i. consent disclosure rules
inframammary
infundibular stalk
infundibuliform hymen
infundibulopelvic ligament
infundibulum
infusion
continuous subcutaneous insulin i.
fetal cortisol i.
intra-arterial i.
intralymphatic i.
intravenous i.
vasopressin i.
ingestion
alcohol i.
inguinal
i. canal
i. hernia
i. lymphadenectomy
i. lymph node
inguinal-femoral node dissection
INH
isoniazid
inhalation
i. anesthesia
smoke i.
inheritance
autosomal dominant i.
autosomal recessive i.
dominant i.
multifactorial i.
polygenic i.

inheritance *(continued)*
- recessive i.
- sex-linked i.

inherited
- i. androgen uptake impairment
- i. disorder
- i. infertility

inhibin

inhibited sexual desire

inhibition
- follicle-stimulating hormone i.
- hemagglutination i.
- labor i.
- luteinization i.
- pituitary gonadotropin i.
- premature uterine contraction i.
- prostaglandin synthesis i.
- steroid secretion i.

inhibitor
- cell growth i.
- cholinesterase i.
- corticotropin-releasing i.
- dihydrofolate reductase i.
- factor VII i.
- follicle-stimulating hormone i.
- follicle stimulating hormone binding i.
- gonadotropin secretion i.
- luteinization i.
- luteinizing hormone receptor binding i.
- monoamine oxidase i.
- oocyte maturation i. (OMI)
- ovum-capture i.
- prostaglandin synthesis i.
- prostaglandin synthetase i. (PGSI)

initiation
- labor i.
- lactation i.
- puberty i.

injectable
- i. bromocriptine
- i. contraception
- i. contraceptive

injection
- adrenaline i.
- continuous subcutaneous insulin i.
- local methotrexate i.
- paracervical i.
- silicone i.
- Teflon periurethral i.

injury
- accidental fetal i.
- birth i.
- brachial plexus i.
- congenital i.
- iatrogenic ureteral i.
- intraoperative gastrointestinal i.
- irradiation i.
- muscular i.
- nerve i.
- obstetrical traction i.
- pelvic nerve i.
- pulmonary i.
- spinal i.
- spinal cord i.
- thermal i.
- traumatic i.
- urological i.
- vaginal i.
- vascular i.

inlet
- pelvic i.

inner cell mass

innominate bone

Innovar

Inocor

inositol trisphosphate

insemination
- artificial i.
- cervical i.
- heterologous i.
- high intrauterine i.
- homologous i.
- intrauterine i.
- i. swim-up technique
- therapeutic i.
- washed intrauterine i.

insensitive
- i. ovary
- i. ovary syndrome

insensitivity
- androgen i.

insertion

insipidus
- diabetes i.

insomnia

inspection

instability
detrusor i.
instillation
instruction
discharge i.'s
instrument
Kevorkian-Younge cervical biopsy i.
insufficiency
adrenal i.
adrenocortical i.
aortic valve i.
corpus luteum i.
mitral valve i.
placental i.
renal i.
uterine i.
uteroplacental i.
insufflation
tubal i.
insulin
maternal i.
i. pump
i. resistance
i. tolerance test
insulinase
insulin-dependent diabetes mellitus (IDDM)
insulin-like growth factor (IGF)
insulin-like growth factor I
intact membrane
Intal
interaction
actin-myosin i.
androgen i.
sperm-oocyte i.
INTERCEED absorbable adhesion barrier
intercourse
sexual i.
interferon (IFN)
alpha i.
alpha-recombinant i.
beta i.
gamma i.
human leukocyte i. (HLI)
leukocyte i.
lymphoblastoid i.
Intergroup Rhabdomyosarcoma Study (IRS)
interleukin (IL)
interleukin-1 (IL-1)
interleukin-1β
interleukin-2 (IL-2)
intermenstrual
i. bleeding
i. pain
intermittent
acute i. porphyria
i. cyclical etidronate disodium
i. hydrosalpinx
i. sterilization
interna
endometriosis i.
internal
i. conjugate
i. endometriosis
i. generative organ
i. genitalia
i. os
i. ovular transmigration
i. podalic version
i. radiation therapy
i. rotation
i. version
internalization
hormone-receptor complex i.
receptor i.
International
I. Association for the Study of Pain
I. Federation of Gynecology and Obstetrics classification
I. Society for Gynecologic Pathology (ISGYP)
I. Society for the Study of Vulvar Diseases (ISSVD)
I. Union Against Cancer (UICC)
international
i. classification of cancer of cervix
interobserver variation
interphase
interpretation
mirror image i.
i. variability
interruption
vena caval i.
intersex problem
interstitial
i. cell
i. ectopic pregnancy

interstitial *(continued)*
- i. and loculated hematoma
- i. mastitis
- i. plasma cell pneumonia
- i. pregnancy
- i. therapy

intertuberous diameter
intervention
- court-ordered obstetrical i.
- legal i.

interventional procedure
intervillous
- i. blood
- i. blood gas
- i. space

intestinal
- i. bypass procedure
- i. conduit
- i. fistula
- i. mesentery
- i. obstruction
- i. parasite
- i. peristalsis
- i. tract

intolerance
- carbohydrate i.
- fructose i.
- gestational carbohydrate i. (GCI)
- glucose i.

intoxication
- water i.

intra-abdominal
- i.-a. pressure
- i.-a. surgery

intra-amniotic infection
intra-arterial infusion
Intrabutazone
intracanalicular fibroadenoma
intracavitary radium
intracellular mediator
intracervical tent
intracranial
- i. anatomy
- i. aneurysm
- i. dural vascular anomaly
- i. hemorrhage
- i. tumor

intracystic papillary carcinoma
intraductal
- i. carcinoma
- i. papillary carcinoma
- i. papilloma

intradural spinal angioma
intraepithelial
- i. cervical dysplasia
- i. disease progression
- i. endometrial cancer
- i. neoplasia
- i. neoplasia of vagina
- i. neoplasia of vulva

intrahepatic cholestasis of pregnancy
intraligamentary pregnancy
intraligamentous myoma
Intralipid
intralobular duct
intralymphatic infusion
intramammary
- i. lymph node

intramural
- i. myoma
- i. myoma of uterus
- i. pregnancy

intranatal
intranuclear virion
intraoperative
- i. gastrointestinal injury
- i. radiation

intrapartum
- i. cardiotocography
- i. hemorrhage
- i. monitoring
- i. period

intraperitoneal
- i. blood transfusion
- i. chemotherapy
- i. cisplatin
- i. cisplatin chemotherapy
- i. endometrial metastatic disease
- i. fetal transfusion
- i. 5-fluorouracil
- i. pregnancy
- i. radiation therapy
- i. therapy

intrauterine
- i. adhesion
- i. amputation
- i. contraceptive device (IUCD)
- i. death
- i. device (IUD)
- i. diaphragm
- i. fetal transfusion
- i. fracture

i. GIFT
i. growth retardation (IUGR)
i. hematoma
i. herpes
i. infection
i. insemination
i. intraperitoneal fetal transfusion
i. pneumonia
i. pregnancy
i. pressure cycle
i. pressure measurement
i. resuscitation
i. synechia
i. transfusion
i. volume

intravaginal
i. cream
i. foam
i. sponge

intravascular transfusion
intravenous
i. alimentation
i. anti-D immunoglobulin
i. drug
i. glucose challenge
i. immunoglobulin
i. infusion
i. leiomyomatosis
i. pyelogram
i. pyelography (IVP)

intraventricular hemorrhage
intravesical pressure
intravillous space
intrinsic
i. dysmenorrhea
i. pulsatility

introitus
Intropin
intubation
endotracheal i.
tracheal i.

invasion
early stromal i.

invasive
i. cancer
i. carcinoma
i. hydatidiform mole
i. mole
i. neoplasia

Inventory
Minnesota Multiphasic Personality I. (MMPI)

inverse square law
Inversine
inversion
i. of chromosomes
paracentric i.
pericentric i.
i. of the uterus

inverted
i. nipple
i. pelvis

investigation
infertility i.

involuntary sterilization
involution
i. cyst
i. of the uterus

involutional
i. melancholia
i. psychosis

involvement
metastatic axillary i.
neurologic i.
ocular i.
pelvic i.

iocetamic acid
iodamide
iodide
potassium i.
sodium i.
i. therapy

iodide-containing medication
iodinated glycerol
iodine
i. douching
i. 125-labeled fibrinogen scan
i. stain
i. supply

iodine-125 (^{125}I)
iodine-131 (^{131}I)
antiferritin antibody linked to i.-131

iodipamide
iodomethyl-norcholesterol scanning
iodoquinol
iodothyronine
ion
calcium i.

Ionamin
ionization

ionizing radiation
iopanoic acid
iothalamate sodium
ipodate sodium
iprindole
iproniazid
^{192}Ir
iridium-192
iridium-192 (^{192}Ir)
iridium wire
iritis
i. catamenialis
IRMA
immunoradiometric assay
iron
i. deficiency anemia
i. requirement
serum i.
irradiation
abdominal i.
abdominopelvic i.
external beam i.
i. injury
local i.
para-aortic node i.
pelvic i.
surface i.
whole-abdomen i.
whole-pelvis i.
irregularity
menstrual i.
irrigation
irritable breast
IRS
Intergroup Rhabdomyosarcoma Study
ischemia
myocardial i.
ischemic heart disease
isethionate
pentamidine i.
ISG
immune serum globulin
ISGYP
International Society for Gynecologic Pathology
island
Langerhans' i.'s
islets of Langerhans
Ismelin
isoamylase
isoantibody
isoantigen
Iso-Bid
isocarboxazid
isochromosome X
isodose curve
isoetharine
isofluorphate
isoflurane
isogeneic graft
isograft
Isohalent Improved
isoimmune thrombocytopenia
isoimmunization
D i.
D-antigen i.
Rh i.
Isolin
isologous neoplasm
isomer
isomerase
triose phosphate i.
isoniazid (INH)
Isopaque
Isophrin
isoprenaline hydrochloride
isopropamide iodide
isoproterenol
Isoptin
Isopto Carbachol
Isopto Carpine
Isopto-Cetamide
Isopto Eserine
Isopto Frin
Isordil
isosorbide dinitrate
Isotamine
isotope
i. scanning
Isotrate
isotretinoin
isovalericacidemia
isoxsuprine hydrochloride
issue
ethical i.
legal i.
social i.
ISSVD
International Society for the Study of Vulvar Diseases
isthmica nodosa
isthmus, pl. **isthmuses, isthmi**
Isuprel
itch-scratch cycle

ITP
immune thrombocytopenic purpura
idiopathic thrombocytopenic purpura

IUCD
intrauterine contraceptive device

IUD
intrauterine device

IUD-related infection

IUGR
intrauterine growth retardation

IVF/ET
in vitro fertilization/embryo transfer

IVP
intravenous pyelography

J

Jackson right angle retractor
Jacobs tenaculum
Janimine
Jarisch-Herxheimer reaction
jaundice
- black j.
- breast milk j.
- cholestatic j.
- j. of the newborn
- physiologic j.

jejunoileal bypass
jello sign
jelly
- contraceptive j.
- Wharton's j.

jeopardy
- fetal j.

Jew
- Ashkenazi J.

jogger's amenorrhea
Johnson's method
joint
- j. deformity
- j. hyperlaxity
- pelvic j.
- sacroiliac j.

Jones and Jones wedge technique
Jorgenson scissors
juice baby
junction
- gap j.
- squamocolumnar j.

justifiable abortion
juvenile
- j. carcinoma
- j. gangliosidosis
- j. papillomatosis
- j. pelvis
- j. rheumatoid arthritis
- j. spermatogonial depletion

K

Kabikinase
Kagan staging system
Kallmann's syndrome
kanamycin
Kantrex
Kaochlor
Kaon
Kaon-Cl
Kaposi's sarcoma
Karmen cannula
Karnofsky
K. performance status of chemotherapy
Kartagener's syndrome
karyopyknotic index
karyotype
fetal k.
45,X k.
46,XX k.
47,XXY k.
46,XY k.
karyotyping
Kasof
Kato
Kay Ciel
Kaylixir
K cell
Keflex
Keflin
Kefzol
Kegel's
K. exercises
Kehr
K. incision
K. technique
Kell sensitization
Kelly
K. clamp
K. plication procedure
K. retractor
Kelly-Gray curette
Kelly's operation
Kemadrin
keratosis
seborrheic k.
kernicterus
ketamine
ketoacidosis
diabetic k.
ketoconazole
3-keto desogestrel
11-ketoetiocholanolone
17-ketogenic steroid
ketonemia
ketonuria
ketoprofen
ketosis
starvation k.
17-ketosteroid
17-k. reductase
ketotic hyperglycemia
kev
kilo-electronvolt
Kevorkian punch biopsy
Kevorkian-Younge
K.-Y. biopsy forceps
K.-Y. cervical biopsy instrument
K.-Y. curette
Keyes
K. dermatologic punch
K. punch
K. punch biopsy
key-in-lock maneuver
Kibrick test
kidney
k. biopsy
cystic k.
k. dialysis
k. disease
k. failure
k. function
k. morphology
pelvic k.
single k.
solitary k.
k. stone
k. transplantation
kidney-derived growth factor
kill
cell k.
log cell k.
killer
k. cell
natural k. cells (NK cells)
kilo-electronvolt (kev)
kinase
myosin light-chain k.
pyruvate k. (PK)
tyrosine k.

kinetics
cell k.
Kjelland-Barton forceps
Kjelland-Luikart forceps
Kjelland's forceps
Klavikordal
Klebsiella
Kleihauer-Betke stain
Klinefelter's syndrome
Klonopin
K-Lor
Klor-Con
Klorvess
Klotrix
Klumpke's
K. palsy
K. paralysis
K-Lyte
knee-chest position
knee-elbow position
knee presentation
knot
false k.'s of umbilical cord
syncytial k.
true k.'s of umbilical cord
Kobayashi vacuum extractor
Kocher clamp
Koch's postulates
koilocytic atypia
koilocytosis
koilocytotic cell
kolpos
Konakion
Korenman's estrogen window hypothesis
Koromex
Krabbe's disease
kraurosis vulvae
Krönig technique
Krukenberg's tumor
K-Tab
Kučera's equation
Kwell
Kwellada
kyphoscoliosis
kyphoscoliotic heart disease
kyphotic pelvis

L

labetalol
labia
labial
l. agglutination
l. fusion
l. hernia
labia majora
labia minora
labioscrotal swelling
labium, pl. **labia**
labor
abnormal l.
active phase of l.
l. augmentation
l. augmentation induction
dry l.
false l.
first stage of l.
induced l.
induced abortion l.
l. inhibition
l. initiation
latent phase of l.
missed l.
oxytocin stimulation of l.
l. pains
precipitate l.
premature l.
preterm l.
prolonged l.
second stage of l.
third stage of l.
l. trial
true l.
laboratory
l. finding
l. test
labyrinthine placenta
laceration
aortic l.
birth canal l.
bladder l.
cervical l.
vaginal l.
β-lactamase-resistant antistaphylococcal antibiotic
lactate
cyclizine l.
l. dehydrogenase (LDH)
lactated
l. Ringer's solution
lactating
l. adenoma
l. breast
lactation
l. amenorrhea
inappropriate l.
l. initiation
l. letdown response
lactational
l. mastitis
lacteal
l. cyst
l. fistula
lactic
l. acid dehydrogenase
l. acidosis
lacticacidemia
lactiferous
l. duct
lactifugal
lactifuge
lactigenous
lactigerous
lactobacillus
Lactobacillus acidophilus
lactocele
lactoflavin
lactogen
human placental l. (HPL)
placental l.
lactorrhea
lactose
lactosuria
lactotropin
lactulose
lacuna, pl. **lacunae**
laetrile
lag
anaphase l.
Lahey
L. forceps
LAK
lymphokine-activated killer cell
lake
subchorial l.
Lamaze method
lamina propria

laminaria
l. tent
lamination
laminin
Langerhans'
L. cells
L. granule
L. islands
islets of L.
Langhans'
L. cells
L. giant cell granuloma
L. stria
Laniazid
Lanophyllin
Lanoxin
Lanvis
laparohysterectomy
laparohystero-oophorectomy
laparohysteropexy
laparohysterosalpingo-oophorectomy
laparohysterotomy
laparomyomectomy
laparosalpingectomy
laparosalpingo-oophorectomy
laparosalpingotomy
laparoscopic
l. cautery
l. electrocautery
l. fenestration
l. management
l. multiple-punch resection
l. salpingostomy
laparoscopy
laser l.
operative l.
pelvic l.
second-look l.
laparotomy
exploratory l.
l. incision
second-look l.
laparotrachelotomy
laparouterotomy
Lapides technique
Largactil
large-for-date infant
Larodopa
laryngeal papillomatosis
laser
l. ablation
l. blanching
carbon dioxide l.
l. cervical conization
l. ejecta
l. laparoscopic management
l. laparoscopy
l. method
Nd:YAG l.
l. photocoagulation
l. photovaporization
l. surgery
l. therapy
l. treatment
Lash's operation
Lasix
last menstrual period (LMP)
late
l. deceleration
l. neonatal death
l. pregnancy
latent
l. herpes simplex virus infection
l. phase of labor
late-onset
l.-o. hydroxylase deficiency
l.-o. hyperplasia
lateral
l. oblique view
l. recumbent position
l. resolution
lateromedial oblique view
lateroversion
latex
l. agglutination
l. particle fixation test
LATS
long-acting thyroid stimulator
LATS-protector
latum
condyloma l.
Latzko's
L. cesarean section
Laufe
L. polyp forceps
Laurence-Moon-Bardet-Biedl syndrome
LAV
lymphadenopathy-associated virus
lavage
peritoneal l.
law
inverse square l.
l. of mass action

Mendel's l.'s
personal injury l.

layer
germ l.
half-value l. (HVL)
Nitabuch's l.

L-Caine

LDH
lactate dehydrogenase

LDL
low-density lipoprotein

LDL-cholesterol

LE
lupus erythematosus

lead

leakage
placental l.
silicone implant l.

***Learning to Eat* manual**

lecithin
disaturated l.

lecithin/sphingomyelin ratio (L/S ratio, L/S ratio)

Ledercillin
L. VK

Lee's report of multiple diverticula

Lee-White method

Le Fort operation

left
l. frontoanterior position (LFA)
l. frontoposterior position (LFP)
l. frontotransverse position (LFT)
l. mentoanterior position (LMA)
l. mentoposterior position (LMP)
l. mentotransverse position (LMT)
l. occipitoanterior position (LOA)
l. occipitoposterior position (LOP)
l. occipitotransverse position (LOT)
l. sacroanterior position (LSA)
l. sacroposterior position (LSP)
l. sacrotransverse position (LST)

left-to-right shunt

leg
l. cramp
l. edema
milk l.
l. thromboembolism
white l.

legal
l. intervention
l. issue
l. status

leg-compression stockings

Legionnaires' disease

leiomyoma, pl. **leiomyomata**
cervical l.
endometrial metastasizing l.
ovarian l.
parasitic l.
submucous l.
leiomyomatata uteri
uterine l.
vascular l.

leiomyomatosis
intravenous l.
l. peritonealis disseminata (LPD)

leiomyosarcoma (LMS)

lemon sign

length
crown-heel l.
crown-rump l.
femur l.

lentivirus

Leopold's maneuvers

leperous salpingitis

leprosy

leptotene stage

Lesch-Nyhan syndrome

lesion
axillary skin l.
barrel-shaped l.
benign l.
benign gynecologic l.
cervical l.
cutaneous l.
genital l.
hyperpigmented l.
lumbosacral plexus l.
lumbosacral root l.
metastatic l.
pigmented l.
plexus l.
precancerous l.

lesion *(continued)*
premalignant l.
radial sclerosing l.
sclerosing l.
skin l.
spiculated l.
vulvar pigmented l.
vulvovaginal l.
LET
linear energy transfer
letdown
milk l.
letdown reflex
lethal dwarfism
leucine aminopeptidase
leucovorin
leukapheresis
leukemia
myelogenous l.
Leukeran
leukocyte
l. count
l. function
l. interferon
l. transfusion
leukocytosis
leukokraurosis
leukomalacia
periventricular l.
leukophlegmasia
l. dolens
leukoplakia
l. vulvae
leukoplakic vulvitis
leukorrhagia
leukorrhea
menstrual l.
leukorrheal
leukotriene
leuprolide acetate
levallorphan tartrate
levamisole
levarterenol
Levate
levator
l. ani
level
amniotic fluid l.
arachidonic acid l.
blood l.
cesium-137 l.
cortisol l.
dynamic test of hormone l.
endogenous estrogen l.
endothelin plasma l.
estriol l.
estrogen l.
fetal LDL l.
gonadotropin l.
hemoglobin l.
hormonal l.
human chorionic gonadotropin l.
human chorionic gonadotropin serum l.
iodothyronine l.
maternal l.
maternal estriol l.
maternal serum l.
peripheral hormone l.
plasma l.
postmenopausal l.
progesterone l.
progesterone myometrial l.
prolactin l.
relaxin serum l.
serum l.
uterine lysosome l.
Levlen
levodopa (L-dopa)
Levo-Dromoran
Levoid
levonorgestrel
Levophed
Levoprome
levorotatory alkaloid
levorphan
levorphanol tartrate
Levothroid
levothyroxine
levoversion
Levret's forceps
Levsin
Levsinex
Leydig
L. cell embryology
L.'s cells
L. cell tumor
LFA
left frontoanterior position
LFP
left frontoposterior position
LFT
left frontotransverse position
LGV
lymphogranuloma venereum

LH
luteinizing hormone
LH Color test
LH-RH
luteinizing hormone-releasing hormone
LH-RH analogue
liability
malpractice l.
libidinal change
libido
decreased l.
Librax
Librium
licentiate in midwifery (L.M.)
lichen
l. planus
l. sclerosus

lichenification
Liddle's test
lidocaine
Lidoject
lie
fetal l.
longitudinal l.
oblique l.
transverse l.
unstable l.
life
l. event
l. expectancy
fetal l.
l. stress
l. table method
l. table survival
wrongful birth and l.
Li-Fraumeni cancer syndrome
ligament
broad l.
cardinal l.
Cooper's l.'s
Cooper's suspensory l.'s
infundibulopelvic l.
Mackenrodt's l.'s
ovarian l.
round l.
transverse cervical l.
triangular l.
umbilical l.
utero-ovarian l.
uterosacral l.
ligamentopexis, ligamentopexy
ligamentum
l. teres
l. venosum
ligase
ligation
bleeding site l.
hypogastric artery l.
modified Irving-type tubal l.
tubal l.
ligature
chromic gut pelviscopic loop l.
lightening
lignocaine
Liley curve
limb
fetal l.
l. motion
l. reduction
limit
confidence l.'s
fetal dose l.
radiation dose l.
limulus amebocyte lysate assay
Lincocin
lincomycin
lindane
line
black l.
iliopectineal l.
multiple resistant cell l.'s
linea, gen. and pl. **lineae**
lineae albicantes
lineae atrophicae
l. nigra
l. terminalis
linear
l. accelerator
l. atrophy
l. energy transfer (LET)
linkage
l. analysis
genetic l.
linoleic acid
Lioresal
liothyronine
liotrix
lip
cleft l.
lipase
lipid
l. cell
l. cell neoplasm

lipid *(continued)*
l. cell ovarian tumor
l. cell tumor
l. metabolism
lipoid
l. adrenal gland hypoplasia
l. adrenal hyperplasia
l. ovarian neoplasm
l. ovarian tumor
lipolysis
lipoma
vulvar l.
lipomatosis
liponecrosis microcystica calcificans
lipoprotein
l. concentration
high-density l. (HDL)
low-density l. (LDL)
very low-density l. (VLDL)
lipoprotein-cholesterol metabolism
liposarcoma
Liposyn
lipotropin
β-lipotropin
μ-lipotropin
Lippes loop
Lippes-type intrauterine device
Lipschütz' ulcer
Liquaemin
liquefaction
semen l.
Liquiprin
liquor folliculi
lisinopril
Lisolipin
Listeria monocytogenes
listeriosis
Lister scissors
Lithane
lithiasis
lithium
Lithobid
Lithonate
lithopedion, lithopedium
Lithotabs
lithotomy
l. position
vaginal l.
litigation
malpractice l.
Litzmann's obliquity
livebirth, live birth
liveborn infant
live poliovirus vaccine
liver
acute fatty l.
cirrhosis of l.
l. disease
fetal l.
l. function test
l. metastasis
l. transplant
l. transplantation
l. tumor
live-virus vaccine
L.M.
licentiate in midwifery
LMA
left mentoanterior position
LMP
last menstrual period
left mentoposterior position
LMS
leiomyosarcoma
LMT
left mentotransverse position
LOA
left occipitoanterior position
lobular
l. carcinoma
l. neoplasia
lobule
local
l. anesthesia
l. anesthetic
l. excision
l. irradiation
l. methotrexate injection
l. ovarian condition
localization
epithelial autoantibody l.
estrogen receptor l.
needle l.
placental l.
location
gene l.
lochia
l. alba
l. cruenta
l. purulenta
l. rubra
l. sanguinolenta
l. serosa
lochial
lochiometra
lochiometritis

lochioperitonitis
lochiorrhagia
lochiorrhea
lock
English l.
French l.
German l.
pivot l.
sliding l.
locked twin
locus, pl. **loci**
genetic l.
Loeb's deciduoma
Loestrin 1.5/30
Loestrin 1/20
Lofene
log cell kill
Lomanate
Lomotil
lomustine
long-acting
l.-a. contraception
l.-a. contraceptive
l.-a. contraceptive steroid
l.-a. thyroid stimulator (LATS)
long arm of chromosome
long-axis view
longitudinal
l. growth
l. lie
l. oval pelvis
l. scan
long-term
l.-t. follow-up
l.-t. sequelae
l.-t. survival
Loniten
Lonox
loop
l. diathermy cervical conization
Lippes l.
low-voltage diathermy l.
somatic nervous system feedback l.
Lo/Ovral
LOP
left occipitoposterior position
loperamide
lophosphamide
Lopressor
Loprox
lorazepam
lordosis
loss
blood l.
bone l.
early embryonic l.
early pregnancy l.
embryonic l.
estrogen l.
excessive blood l.
hair l.
heat l.
menstrual blood l.
normal blood l.
postmenopausal bone l.
pregnancy l.
rapid bone l.
recurrent pregnancy l.
repetitive pregnancy l.
spinal bone l.
surgical weight l.
vertebral bone l.
water l.
weight l.
LOT
left occipitotransverse position
louse, pl. **lice**
crab l.
low
l. birth weight
l. cervical cesarean section
l. forceps
l. hematocrit
l. intrafollicular 17β-estradiol
l. platelets
l. rectal resection
l. steroid content combined oral contraceptive
l. vesicovaginal fistula
low-back pain
low-birth-weight infant
low-density lipoprotein (LDL)
low-dose
l.-d. danazol
l.-d. heparin
l.-d. oral contraceptive
lower
l. abdominal pain
l. abdominal tenderness
l. extremity
l. genital tract infection
l. limb ossification center

lower *(continued)*
l. urinary tract
l. urinary tract infection
l. uterine segment
lower-segment scar
low-residue diet
low-segment transverse incision
low-voltage diathermy loop
loxapine
Loxitane
Lozol
L-PAM
melphalan
LPD
leiomyomatosis peritonealis disseminata
LSA
left sacroanterior position
LSD
lysergic acid diethylamide
LSP
left sacroposterior position
L/S ratio
lecithin/sphingomyelin ratio
LST
left sacrotransverse position
lubricant
vaginal l.
Lub's syndrome
Lucite dilator
Ludiomil
Lugol's
L. iodine solution
Luikart forceps
Lumadex-FSI test
lumbar
l. artery
l. epidural anesthesia
lumbosacral
l. intervertebral disk abnormality
l. plexus lesion
l. root lesion
Luminal
Lumopaque
lump
lumpectomy
lung
l. cancer
l. capacity
l. carcinoma
l. compliance
l. edema
hypoplastic l.
l. profile
l. volume
Lupron
lupus
l. anticoagulant
l. anticoagulant activity
l. anticoagulant antibody
l. crisis
l. erythematosus (LE)
l. obstetric syndrome
luteal
l. function
l. ovarian cyst
l. phase
l. phase defect
l. phase inadequacy
lutein cell
luteinization
l. inhibition
l. inhibitor
l. stimulator
luteinized
l. follicle
l. thecoma
l. unruptured follicle
l. unruptured follicle syndrome
luteinizing
l. hormone (LH)
l. hormone hypersecretion
l. hormone receptor binding inhibitor
l. hormone-releasing hormone (LH-RH)
l. hormone-releasing hormone analogue
l. hormone secretion
luteinoma
luteolysis
luteolytic
l. action
luteoma
pregnancy l.
luteoplacental shift
luteum
corpus l.
Lyme disease
lymph
l. node
l. node drainage
l. node endometriotic adenoacanthoma

l. node metastasis
l. node positivity
lymphadenectomy
inguinal l.
Meigs pelvic l.
pelvic l.
retroperitoneal l.
lymphadenitis
mesenteric l.
lymphadenopathy
axillary l.
lymphadenopathy-associated virus (LAV)
lymphangiography
lymphangioma
lymphatic
l. drainage
lymphatics
paracervical l.
lymphedema
lymphoblastoid interferon
lymphocyst
lymphocyte
l. activator
B l.
l. dysfunction
l. immune response
natural killer l.
T l.
T_4 l.
lymphocyte-activating factor
lymphocytic
l. adenohypophysitis
lymphogranuloma
l. inguinale
venereal l., l. venereum
lymphography
lymphoid
l. cell
l. hypophysitis
l. tissue
lymphokine
lymphokine-activated
l.-a. killer cell (LAK)
lymphoma
malignant l.
metastatic l.
non-Hodgkin's l.
ovarian l.
recurrent l.
lymphosarcoma
lymphotoxin antitumor activity
lynestrenol
Lyon hypothesis
lypressin
lysergic
l. acid
l. acid diethylamide (LSD)
lysine
lysis
adhesion l.
lysosomal
l. acid phosphatase
l. acid phosphate
l. enzyme disorder
lysosome

M

M
M antigen
M phase
mitosis phase
maceration
fetal m.
Mach band effect
MAC/HC ratio
machine
cobalt megavoltage m.
megavoltage m.
Mackenrodt's ligaments
macroadenoma
prolactin-secreting m.
macrocytic anemia of pregnancy
Macrodantin
α_2-macroglobulin
macromastia, macromazia
macrophage
m. colony-stimulating factor
macrophage-activating factor (MAF)
macrophage-inhibition factor
macroprolactinoma
macrosomia
fetal m.
Madlener operation
MAF
macrophage-activating factor
mafenide
Magan
magma reticulare
magnesia
milk of m.
magnesium
m. citrate
m. hydroxide
m. salicylate
m. sulfate
magnetically responsive microsphere
magnetic resonance imaging (MRI)
magnetite (Fe_3O_4)
m. in tumor targeting
magnification
m. mammography
spot m.
Magrina-Bookwalter vaginal retractor
maidenhead
major
m. histocompatibility antigen
β-thalassemia m.
malabsorption
congenital folate m.
malacoplakia
malaria
male
m. factor
m. factor infertility
m. fertility
m. genital duct
m. genital duct development
m. infertility
m. pseudohermaphroditism
m. puberty
m. reproductive system
m. sex differentiation
m. sterility
m. sterilization
46,XX m.
maleate
ergonovine m.
methylergonovine m.
methysergide m.
malformation
arteriovenous m.
clomiphene fetal m.
congenital m.
fetal m.
m. rate
malignancy
extrapelvic m.
gastrointestinal m.
genital tract m.
vulvar m.
malignant
m. calcification
m. cytotrophoblast
m. degeneration
m. effusion
m. lymphoma
m. melanoma
m. mixed müllerian tumor (MMMT)
m. neoplasm
m. ovarian neoplasm
m. ovarian teratoma
m. ovarian tumor

malignant *(continued)*
m. pleural effusion
m. syncytiotrophoblast
m. teratoma
m. tumor of cervix
malignum
adenoma m.
malleable retractor
Malmström vacuum extractor
malnutrition
Malotuss
malposition
uterine m.
malpractice
m. claim
m. liability
m. litigation
m. suit
malpresentation
mamma, gen. and pl. **mammae**
m. accessoria
m. erratica
supernumerary m.
mammalgia
mammaplasty, mammoplasty
augmentation m.
reconstructive m.
reduction m.
mammary
m. calculus
m. duct ectasia
m. dysplasia
m. fistula
m. gland
m. neuralgia
m. souffle
mammectomy
mammillaplasty
mammillitis
mammitis
mammogram
mammographic
m. detection
m. screening
mammography
magnification m.
mammose
mammotomy
mammotropic, mammotrophic
mAMSA
Amsacrine
management
active third-stage m.
epilepsy m.
expectant m.
infertility m.
laparoscopic m.
laser laparoscopic m.
metabolic m.
noninvasive m.
physiologic third-stage m.
pregnancy m.
preoperative m.
risk m.
surgical m.
Manchester
M. operation
M. ovoid
M. system for radium therapy
Manchester-Fothergil operation
Mandelamine
mandelic acid
Mandelurine
mandible
Mandol
maneuver
Bill's m.
Bracht m.
Brandt-Andrews m.
Credé's m.'s
DeLee's m.
forceps m.
Hillis-Müller m.
key-in-lock m.
Leopold's m.'s
Mauriceau-Levret m.
Mauriceau's m.
McDonald's m.
McRoberts m.
midforceps m.
Pajot's m.
Pinard's m.
Prague m.
Ritgen's m.
Rubin's m.
Scanzoni's m.
Scanzoni-Smellie m.
Sellick's m.
Wigand m.
Woods' screw m.
manifestation
ocular m.
renal m.
manipulation
gamete m.

Mann isthmic cerclage
mannitol
mannosidosis
manual
Learning to Eat m.
m. pelvimetry
m. rotation
map
gene m.
maple syrup urine disease
mapping
gene m.
maprotiline
Marañón's syndrome
Marchand's
M. adrenals
M. rest
Marchetti test
Marezine
Marfan's syndrome
Margesic A-C
marginal sinus rupture
marijuana
m. effect
marker
adrenal hyperandrogenism m.
assay m.
DNA m.
m. gene
genetic m.
peripheral androgen activity m.
tumor m.
Marlex
Marmine
Maroteaux-Lamy syndrome
Marplan
marrow
bone m.
Marshall-Marchetti-Krantz operation
marsupialization
Spence and Duckett m.
m. technique
transurethral m.
Martius
M. procedure
M. procedure-bulbocavernosus fat flap
masculine pelvis
masculinization
masculinovoblastoma
mask
m. of pregnancy
ventilation by m.
mass
adnexal m.
benign m.
bleeder in tumor m.
bone m.
circumscribed m.
cortical m.
cystic adnexal m.
fallopian tube m.
ill-defined m.
inner cell m.
mixed-density m.
noncalcified nodular m.
ovarian m.
pelvic m.
persistent ovarian m.
postmenopausal body m.
stellate m.
tubal m.
tumor m.
uterine m.
vertebral bone m.
well-defined m.
massage
cardiac m.
closed chest m.
uterine m.
massive
m. breast hypertrophy
m. ovarian cyst
m. transfusion
mastadenitis
mastadenoma
mastalgia
mastatrophy, mastatrophia
mastectomy
extended radical m.
modified radical m.
radical m.
simple m.
subcutaneous m.
total m.
mastitis
chronic cystic m.
gargantuan m.
glandular m.
granulomatous m.
interstitial m.
lactational m.
m. neonatorum

mastitis *(continued)*
- parenchymatous m.
- phlegmonous m.
- plasma cell m.
- puerperal m.
- retromammary m.
- stagnation m.
- submammary m.
- suppurative m.

mastodynia
mastoncus
mastopathy
mastopexy
mastoplasia
mastoplasty
mastoptosis
mastorrhagia
mastoscirrhus
mastotomy
material
- genetic m.
- metal suture m.
- nylon suture m.
- polyester suture m.
- polyethylene suture m.
- polypropylene suture m.
- radiocontrast m.
- suture m.
- synthetic suture m.

maternal
- m. abdominal pressure
- m. age
- m. alcohol consumption
- m. alcoholism
- m. anesthesia
- m. antibody
- m. aspirin use
- m. asthma
- m. attitude
- m. birthing position
- m. blood
- m. blood study
- m. cholestasis
- m. coagulopathy
- m. cocaine abuse
- m. cocaine use
- m. condition
- m. cortical vein
- m. cortical vein thrombosis
- m. cotyledon
- m. cyanotic heart disease
- m. death
- m. death rate
- m. diabetes
- m. disease
- m. douching
- m. drug abuse
- m. dystocia
- m. estriol level
- m. exercise
- m. factor
- m. febrile morbidity
- m. fracture
- m. gonad
- m. hepatitis
- m. HLA haplotype
- m. hydration
- m. hydrops
- m. hydrops syndrome
- m. hyperparathyroidism
- m. hypertension
- m. hypotension
- m. immune response
- m. immunology
- m. infection
- m. insulin
- m. mercury exposure
- m. morbidity
- m. mortality
- m. mortality rate
- m. nutrition
- m. ocular adaptation
- m. outcome
- m. Parvovirus fetalis
- m. peripheral blood
- m. phenylketonuria
- m. physiology
- m. platelet
- m. position
- m. pulse
- m. pyrexia
- m. risk
- m. screening
- m. serum
- m. serum alpha-fetoprotein (MSAFP)
- m. serum alpha-fetoprotein level
- m. serum level
- m. size
- m. smoking
- m. stature
- m. steroid concentration
- m. stress
- m. surgery
- m. surveillance

m. thrombocytopenia
m. tissue
m. trauma
m. undernourishment
m. vascular response
m. weight
maternal-fetal
m.-f. histoincompatibility
m.-f. HLA compatibility
m.-f. transmission
maternal-placental-fetal unit
maternal-placental unit
maternity
disputed m.
matter
particulate m.
maturation
fetal lung m.
follicular m.
ovum m.
pulmonary m.
skeletal m.
m. value
mature
m. cystic ovarian teratoma
m. ovarian teratoma
maturity
fetal m.
fetal lung m.
fetal pulmonary m.
Mauriceau-Levret maneuver
Mauriceau's maneuver
Maxeran
maximal permissible dose
maximum breathing capacity
Maxolon
Mayer-Rokitansky-Küster-Hauser syndrome
Mayer's pessary
Maylard incision
Mayo
M. curved scissors
M. scissors
M. straight scissors
Mayo-Hegar needle holder
Mazanor
mazindol
mazodynia
mazolysis
mazopathy, mazopathia
mazopexy
mazoplasia
MBP
modified Bagshawe protocol
McCall stitch
McCune-Albright syndrome
McDonald
M. cervical cerclage
M. procedure
McDonald's maneuver
McIndoe's operation
McKusick-Kaufman syndrome
McLean forceps
MCR
metabolic clearance rate
McRoberts maneuver
Meadows' syndrome
mean
m. hemoglobin concentration
m. menstrual cycle hematocrit
m. plasma iron concentration
regression to m.
measles
German m.
m. vaccine
measurement
acid-base m.
fetal growth m.
intrauterine pressure m.
optical density m.
transcutaneous m.
Measurin
mebanazine
Mebaral
Mebendacin
mebendazole
Mebutar
mecamylamine
mechanical dysmenorrhea
mechanism
alloimmune m.
autoimmune m.
cellular cytotoxic m.
Douglas' m.
Duncan's m.
heat transfer m.
host defense m.
host response m.
Schultze's m.
two-cell m.
mechlorethamine
meclizine hydrochloride

meclofenamate
Meclomen
mecometer
meconial colic
meconiorrhea
meconium
m. aspiration
m. aspiration syndrome
m. blockage syndrome
m. ileus
m. ileus appearance
m. peritonitis
m. plug
m. stain
m. staining
medial oblique view
median
m. eminence
m. episiotomy
mediating action
mediator
intracellular m.
medical
m. ethics
m. history
m. record
medication
iodide-containing m.
over-the-counter m.
medicine
fetal m.
neonatal m.
perinatal m.
space m.
medicolegal aspects
Medihaler-Epi
Medihaler-Iso
Medilium
mediolateral
m. episiotomy
m. view
Meditran
medium
transmission m.
medorrhea
medroxyprogesterone
m. acetate (MPA)
medulla oblongata
medullary carcinoma
mefenamic acid
Mefoxin
Megace
megacolon
toxic m.
megaloblastic anemia
megavolt (Mev)
megavoltage machine
megestrol acetate
meglumine diatrizoate
Meigs-Okabayashi procedure
Meigs pelvic lymphadenectomy
Meigs' syndrome
Meigs-Werthein hysterectomy
meiosis
diakinesis stage of oocyte m.
dictyate stage of oocyte m.
oocyte m.
melancholia
involutional m.
melanocyte-stimulating hormone
melanocytic nevus
melanoma
Clark classification of vulvar m.
cutaneous m.
malignant m.
metastatic m.
nodular m.
superficial spreading m.
vulvar m.
melasma
m. gravidarum
melatonin
m. secretion
Melfiat
Mellaril
mellitus
diabetes m.
insulin-dependent diabetes m. (IDDM)
non-insulin-dependent diabetes m. (NIDDM)
overt insulin-dependent diabetes m.
melphalan (L-PAM)
membrana granulosa
membrane
dysmenorrheal m.
erythrocyte m.
exocelomic m.
extraembryonic fetal m.
fetal m.
Heuser's m.
intact m.

mucous m.'s
placental m.
premature rupture of m. (PROM)
preterm rupture of m.
m. rupture
ruptured m.
spontaneous rupture of m.
vitelline m.

membranous
m. dysmenorrhea
m. glomerulonephritis
m. twin

memory
m. cell
m. phenomenon

menacme

menadiol
m. sodium diphosphate

menadione

menarche
delayed m.

menarcheal, menarchial

mendelian
m. disorder
m. trait

Mendel's laws

Mendelson's syndrome

Menest

Menge's pessary

meningitis, pl. **meningitides**

meningococcal
m. polysaccharide vaccine

meningococcus vaccine

meningoencephalocele

meningomyelocele

Menkes' syndrome

menocelis

menometrorrhagia

menopausal
m. estrogen replacement therapy
m. syndrome

menopause
iatrogenic m.
premature m.

menophania

menorrhagia

menorrhalgia

menoschesis

menostasis, menostasia

menostaxis

menotropin

menouria

menoxenia

menses

menstrual
m. age
m. aspiration
m. blood loss
m. colic
m. cycle
m. cycle induction
m. cycle regulation
m. cycle resumption
m. edema
m. endometrium
m. extraction
m. extraction abortion
m. formula
m. history
m. irregularity
m. leukorrhea
m. molimina
m. period
m. reflux
m. sclerosis
m. state

menstrual-ovarian cycle

menstruant

menstruate

menstruation
abnormal m.
anovular m.
delayed m.
retained m.
retrograde m.
supplementary m.
suppressed m.
vicarious m.

mental
m. development
m. disturbance
m. retardation
m. status evaluation

mentoanterior position

mentoposterior position

mentotransverse position

mentum, gen. **menti**
m. anterior presentation
m. posterior presentation

mepenzolate bromide

meperidine hydrochloride

mephentermine

mephenytoin

mephobarbital

Mephyton
mepindolol
meprobamate
Meprospan
mepyramine
MER
methanol extraction residue
meralgia paraesthetica
2-mercaptoethane sulfonate (MESNA)
mercaptopurine
6-mercaptopurine
Mersilene
M. fascial strip
M. mesh
M. suture
Meruvax II
Mesantoin
mesatipellic pelvis
mesenchyme
nonspecific m.
mesenteric
m. artery
m. lymphadenitis
mesentery
intestinal m.
mesh
Mersilene m.
MESNA
2-mercaptoethane sulfonate
mesoderm
mesodermal sarcoma
mesometanephric carcinoma
mesometric pregnancy
mesometritis
meson
negative π m.
mesonephric
m. adenocarcinoma
m. carcinoma
m. duct
m. rest
m. tubule
mesonephroid tumor
mesonephroma
mesonephros, pl. **mesonephroi**
mesoridazine besylate
mesosalpinx
mesothelioma
benign m. of genital tract
mesovarium, pl. **mesovaria**
messenger
m. RNA (mRNA)
second m.
Mestinon
mestranol
mesylate
2-Br-alpha-ergocryptine m.
dihydroergotamine m.
metabolic
m. acidemia
m. acidosis
m. clearance rate (MCR)
m. disorder
m. error
m. management
metabolism
aerobic m.
amino acid m.
carbohydrate m.
estrogen m.
fat m.
fetal m.
inborn errors of m.
m. in intraperitoneal chemotherapy
lipid m.
lipoprotein-cholesterol m.
mineral m.
neonatal m.
progesterone m.
prostaglandin m.
steroid m.
vitamin m.
water m.
metabolite
steroid m.
metacyesis
Metahydrin
metal
m. coil
m. metabolism disorder
m. suture material
trace m.
metallic bead chain cystourethrography
metanephric duct
metanephros, pl. **metanephroi**
metaphase
metaplasia
ciliated m.
coelomic m.
squamous m.
squamous m. of amnion

tubal m.
vaginal squamous m.
metaplastic carcinoma
Metaprel
metaproterenol sulfate
metaraminol bitartrate
metastasis, pl. **metastases**
adnexal m.
aortic node m.
bony m.
fallopian tube m.
floxuridine in hepatic m.
hepatic m.
inguinal lymph node m.
liver m.
lymph node m.
ovarian m.
ovarian cancer m.
placental m.
pulmonary m.
stomach cancer m.
uterine sarcoma m.
vascular m.
metastatic
m. adenocarcinoma
m. axillary involvement
m. carcinoma
m. lesion
m. lymphoma
m. melanoma
met-enkephalin
meter
glucose m.
metergoline
methacycline hydrochloride
methadone hydrochloride
methamphetamine hydrochloride
m. h. exposure
methandrostenolone
methanol extraction residue (MER)
methantheline bromide
methaqualone
metharbital
methazolamide
methdilazine hydrochloride
methenamine
Methergine
methicillin sodium
methimazole
methixene hydrochloride
method
Billings m.
cold knife m.
contraceptive m.
Credé's m.'s
Johnson's m.
Lamaze m.
laser m.
Lee-White m.
life table m.
rhythm m.
Stroganoff's m.
sympto-thermal m.
methotrexate
methotrimeprazine
methoxamine hydrochloride
methoxyflurane
methoxyphenamine hydrochloride
methscopolamine
methsuximide
methyclothiazide
methylbromide
hyoscine m.
scopolamine m.
methyl-CCNU
methyldopa
methylene blue
methylergometrine maleate
methylergonovine maleate
methylmalonic
m. acidemia
m. aciduria
methylmercury
methylphenidate hydrochloride
methylprednisolone
m. allergic reaction
15-methyl prostaglandin $F_{2\alpha}$
α-methyl-*p*-tyrosine
methyltestosterone
methylxanthine
methysergide maleate
metoclopramide hydrochloride
metolazone
metoprolol
Metra
metratonia
metratrophy, metratrophia
metria
metritis
metrizamide
metrizoate sodium
Metrodin
metrodynamometer
metrodynia
metrography
metrolymphangitis

metromalacia
metromalacoma, metromalacosis
metronidazole
metroparalysis
metropathia
m. hemorrhagica
metropathic
metropathy
metroperitoneal fistula
metroperitonitis
metrophlebitis
metroplasty
Strassman m.
metrorrhagia
m. myopathica
metrorrhea
metrorrhexis
metrosalpingitis
metrosalpingography
metroscope
metrostaxis
metrostenosis
metrotomy
metyrapone test
metyrosine
Metz
Metzenbaum
Metzenbaum (Metz)
M. long scissors
M. scissors
Mev
megavolt
mexiletine
Mexitil
MHA
microhemagglutination assay
Micatin
miconazole nitrate
microadenoma
microangiopathic hemolysis
microangiopathy
thrombotic m.
microatelectasis
microbial
m. factor
m. flora
microbiology
microcalcification
microcephaly
microcyst
milk of calcium m.
microcystica
microencephaly
microenvironment
microfibrillar collagen
microflora
vaginal m.
microglandular
m. adenosis
m. cervical hyperplasia
microhemagglutination
m. assay (MHA)
microhysteroscope
microinjection
microinvasion
stromal m.
microinvasive
m. carcinoma
m. carcinoma classification
m. cervical cancer
m. cervical carcinoma
m. vulvar carcinoma
micromazia
micronized
m. estradiol
m. progesterone
Micronor
microscopy
dark-field m.
microsphere
magnetically responsive m.
Microsulfon
microsurgery
distal tubal m.
tubal m.
tubocornual m.
microsurgical tubocornual anastomosis
microthelia
MicroTrak test
microviscometry
micturition
Midamor
midarm circumference
midcycle
m. cervical mucus
m. surge
middle
m. pain
m. sacral artery
midforceps
m. delivery
m. maneuver
m. operation
midline incision
midmenstrual

midodrine
midpain
midpelvis
midplane
midstream urine specimen
midwife
midwifery
licentiate in m. (L.M.)
MIF
migration-inhibitory factor
mifepristone
migraine
m. headache
migration
cellular m.
placental m.
migration-inhibitory factor (MIF)
mild endometriosis
Milex cervical cup
miliaria
apocrine m.
milk
breast m.
m. of calcium microcyst
cow's m.
m. cyst
m. ejection
m. fever
m. leg
m. letdown
m. of magnesia
uterine m.
witch's m.
Miller-Abbott tube
Miller-Dieker syndrome
mill wheel murmur
Milontin
Miltown
β-mimetic
Minamata disease
mineral
m. metabolism
m. oil
m. requirement
mineralocorticoid
m. production
mineralocorticosteroid
minidose heparin
mini-heparin
minilaparotomy
minimal-incision pubovaginal suspension
Minims
minimum lethal dose (MLD)
mini-pill
Minipress
Minizide
Minnesota Multiphasic Personality Inventory (MMPI)
Minocin
minocycline
minor
α-thalassemia m.
β-thalassemia m.
minoxidil
Mintezol
minute
m. oxygen uptake
m. ventilatory volume
Minzolum
Miocarpine
Miostat
Miradon
mirror image interpretation
miscarriage
recurrent m.
threatened m.
miscarry
mismatch
ventilation/perfusion m.
misonidazole
missed
m. abortion
m. labor
m. period
Mist
Bronitin M.
Mithracin
mithramycin
mitogen
pokeweed m. (PWM)
mitogenic activity
mitomycin
m. C
mitosis
m. phase (M phase)
mitotic figure
mitoxantrone
mitral
m. commissurotomy
m. prolapse
m. regurgitation
m. stenosis
m. valve
m. valve insufficiency

mitral *(continued)*
m. valve prolapse
m. valve stenosis
Mittelschmerz
Mityvac vacuum extractor
mixed
m. connective-tissue disease
m. germ cell tumor
m. gonadal dysgenesis
m. lymphocyte reaction blocking factor
m. mesodermal sarcoma (MMS)
m. mesodermal tumor
m. müllerian sarcoma
m. ovarian mesodermal sarcoma
m. umbilical arterial acidemia
m. uterine tumor
mixed-density mass
Miya hook ligature carrier
MLD
minimum lethal dose
MMMT
malignant mixed müllerian tumor
M-mode ultrasound
MMPI
Minnesota Multiphasic Personality Inventory
MMS
mixed mesodermal sarcoma
MOA
monoamine oxidase
Moban
Mobenol
Mobidin
mobility
bladder neck m.
Modane
M. Soft
mode
delivery m.
Modecate
model
diagnostic m.
Model Uniform Parentage Act
ModiCon
modification
Goodall-Power m.
modified
m. Bagshawe protocol (MBP)
m. Irving-type tubal ligation
m. Pomeroy technique
m. radical hysterectomy
m. radical mastectomy
modifier
biologic response m. (BRM)
Moditen
modulation
antigenic m.
sex steroid m.
mogen clamp
molar
m. degeneration
m. pregnancy
Molatoc
mold
mole
amniography in hydatidiform m.
blood m.
Breus m.
carneous m.
complete hydatidiform m.
cystic m.
false m.
fleshy m.
grape m.
hydatidiform m., hydatid m.
invasive m.
invasive hydatidiform m.
partial hydatidiform m.
tuberous m.
vesicular m.
vulvar hydatidiform m.
molecular
m. analysis
m. clone
m. genetic analysis
m. genetic technique
molestation
sexual m.
molimen, pl. **molimina**
menstrual molimina
molindone
molluscum
m. contagiosum
m. fibrosum gravidarum
molybdenum target
Mondor's disease

mongolism
Monilia
monilial vaginitis
Monistat
monitor
electronic fetal m.
monitoring
blood sugar m.
critical care m.
electronic fetal m.
fetal m.
fetal heart rate m.
heart rate m.
hemodynamic m.
intrapartum m.
tactile sensory m.
monoamine
m. oxidase (MOA)
m. oxidase inhibitor
monoamniotic
monobactam
monochorionic
m. diamniotic placenta
m. monoamniotic
m. monoamniotic placenta
Monocid
monoclonal
m. antibody
monocyte
monodermal tumor
monogamy
mononeuropathy
peripheral m.
monophosphate
adenosine m. (AMP)
cyclic adenosine m. (cAMP)
cytidine m.
monosomy
autosomal m.
m. X
monosymptomatic delusional pseudocyesis
monozygotic twins
Monsel's solution
mons pubis
Montgomery's
M. glands
M. tubercles
mood state
morbidity
fetal m.
infant m.
maternal m.
maternal febrile m.
neonatal m.
perinatal m.
m. predictor
puerperal m.
morcellation
Morgagni
hydatid cyst of M.
Morgagni's tubercle
Morganella
morning
m. sickness
m. vomiting
morning-after pill
morphine
epidural m.
morphological characteristic
morphology
adrenal gland m.
endometrial m.
kidney m.
mortality
m. data
fetal m.
high altitude perinatal m.
infant m.
maternal m.
neonatal m.
perinatal m.
m. predictor
prenatal m.
m. rate
reproductive m.
m. risk factor
morula
mosaicism
mosaic pattern
mother
diabetic m.
D^u-positive m.
high-risk m.
hysterical m.
infant of diabetic m.
surrogate m.
mother-child contact
motherhood
surrogate m.
moth patch
motilin
motion
early cardiac m.
fetal cardiac m.
limb m.

Motrin
mould
mount
wet m.
mouse
hypogonadal m.
nude m.
movement
cardinal m.'s
fetal m.
fetal body m.
rapid eye m. (REM)
sound-stimulated fetal m.
moxalactam
Moxam
MPA
medroxyprogesterone acetate
MRI
magnetic resonance imaging
mRNA
messenger RNA
MSAFP
maternal serum alpha-fetoprotein
mucinous
m. adenocarcinoma of ovary
m. carcinoma
m. cystadenocarcinoma
m. cystadenoma of ovary
m. endometrial carcinoma
m. ovarian neoplasm
m. tumor
mucocolpos
mucoid myoma degeneration
mucopolysaccharidosis
mucopurulent cervicitis
mucorrhea
cervical m.
mucosa
endocervical m.
vaginal m.
mucous
m. membranes
m. plug
mucus
cervical m.
midcycle cervical m.
mulberry ovary
müllerian
m. abnormality
m. adenosarcoma
m. agenesis
m. anomaly
m. cyst
m. duct
m. fusion
m. hypoplasia
m. regression factor
m. sarcoma of uterus
müllerian-inhibiting substance
Müller's tubercle
multicentric carcinoma
multichannel recorder
multifactorial inheritance
multifetal pregnancy
multifetation
multifollicular ovary
multigravida
multilocular cyst
multimammae
multinucleation parakeratosis
multipara
grand m.
multiparity
grand m.
multiparous
multiple
m. birth
m. cervix
m. cyst
m. gestation
m. myeloma
m. organ failure
m. pregnancy
m. resistant cell lines
m. sclerosis
multiple-punch resection
multivariate analysis
multivitamin
mumps
m. vaccine
m. virus
Mumpsvax
mural pregnancy
Murless
M. head extractor
M. head retractor
murmur
mill wheel m.
systolic m.
muscle
bulbocavernosus m.
detrusor m.
gracilis m.
iliococcygeal m.

levator ani m.
pectoralis major m.
pubococcygeal m.
puborectal m.
m. relaxant
smooth m.
m. splitting
striated m.
muscular
m. dystrophy
m. injury
musculoskeletal
mustard
nitrogen m.
phenylalanine m.
L-phenylalanine m.
Mustargen
Mutamycin
mutant cell
mutation
gene m.
point m.
myalgia
Myambutol
myasthenia gravis
Mycelex
Mycifradin
Myciguent
Mycobacterium
M. leprae
Mycoplasma
M. hominis
M. pneumoniae
mycoplasma
genital m.
Mycostatin
mycotic vaginosis
myelocele
myelogenous leukemia
myelography
myeloma
multiple m.
m. protein
myelomeningocele
myelosuppressive agent
Myleran
Mylicon
myoblastoma
granular cell m.
myocardial
m. blood flow
m. function
m. hypertrophy
m. infarction
m. ischemia
Myochrysine
myocolpitis
myocutaneous flap
myoepithelial cell
myoma
asymptomatic m.
cervical m.
degenerating m.
intraligamentous m.
intramural m.
parasitic m.
submucosal m.
submucous m.
subserosal m.
subserous m.
uterine m.
myomata uteri
myomectomy
abdominal m.
vaginal m.
myometrial contraction
myometritis
myometrium
hypotonic m.
uterine m.
myomotomy
myonecrosis
myosalpingitis
myosalpinx
myosin
m. filament
m. light-chain kinase
m. light-chain phosphorylation
myotonia
m. congenita
m. neonatorum
myotonic dystrophy
myrtiform caruncle
Mysoline
Mytelase
myxorrhea

N

nabothian
n. cyst
n. follicle
nadolol
Nadopen-V
Nadrothyron-D
Naegele forceps
nafarelin acetate
nafazatin
Nafcil
nafcillin
Nägele's
N. obliquity
N. rule
nalbuphine
n. hydrochloride
Nalcrom
Nalfon
Nal-Glu
nalidixic acid
nalorphine
naloxone hydrochloride
naltrexone
Naprosyn
naproxen
Naqua
Narcan
narcotic
n. analgesia
n. analgesic
n. antagonist
n. depression
Nardil
nasal
Allerest n.
Coricidin n.
nasogastric tube
nasopharyngeal suction
natal
natality
natimortality
National
N. Collaborative Diethylstilbestrol Adenosis Project (DESAD)
N. Institutes of Health Consensus Conference
N. Surgical Adjuvant Breast Project (NSABP)
native squamous epithelium
natural
n. antibody
n. childbirth
n. conception
n. family planning
n. killer cells (NK cells)
n. killer lymphocyte
Naturetin
nausea
n. gravidarum
n. and vomiting
Navane
Naxen
Nd:YAG
neodymium:yytrium-aluminum garnet
Nd:YAG laser
near-term pregnancy
Nebcin
neck
bladder n.
necrosis
acute tubular n.
cortical n.
fascial n.
fat n.
hepatic n.
periportal hemorrhagic n.
pituitary n.
postsurgical fat n.
posttraumatic fat n.
renal cortical n.
renal tubular n.
uterine n.
necrotizing
n. enterocolitis
n. fasciitis
needle
n. aspiration
n. biopsy
n. localization
negative π meson
NegGram
negligence
Neisseria gonorrhoeae
neisserial infection
nem
Nemasole
Nembutal
Neo-Codema

neodymium:yytrium-aluminum garnet (Nd:YAG)
NeoFed
neogala
neomycin
neonatal
n. condition
n. conjunctivitis
n. death
n. diagnosis
n. distress
n. encephalopathy
n. HSV-1 encephalitis
n. HSV-2 encephalitis
n. hypocalcemia
n. hypoglycemia
n. infection
n. intraventricular hemorrhage
n. medicine
n. metabolism
n. morbidity
n. mortality
n. mortality rate
n. ocular prophylaxis
n. outcome
n. ovary
n. respiratory distress syndrome
n. resuscitation
n. sepsis
n. tetany
neonate
preterm n.
neonatologist
neonatology
neonatorum
ophthalmia n.
Neopap
neoplasia
cervical n.
cervical epithelial n.
cervical intraepithelial n. (CIN)
endometrial n.
endometrial intraepithelial n. (EIN)
gestational trophoblastic n. (GTN)
hematologic n.
intraepithelial n.
invasive n.
lobular n.
thyroid n.
trophoblastic n.
vaginal intraepithelial n. (VAIN)
vulvar intraepithelial n. (VIN)
neoplasm
adrenal n.
benign ovarian n.
bilateral ovarian n.
borderline epithelial ovarian n.
borderline malignant epithelial n.
epithelial stromal ovarian n.
germ cell ovarian n.
hepatic n.
indigenous n.
isologous n.
large intestine n.
lipid cell n.
lipoid ovarian n.
malignant n.
malignant ovarian n.
mucinous ovarian n.
ovarian n.
ovarian lipid cell n.
ovarian malignant epithelial n.
serous ovarian n.
sex cord stromal n.
sex cord-stromal ovarian n.
soft-tissue ovarian n.
neoplastic
n. sequela
n. trophoblastic disease
neosalpingostomy
terminal n.
neostigmine
Neo-Synephrine
neovagina
nephrectomy
nephritis, pl. **nephritides**
n. gravidarum
nephrogenic cord
nephrolithiasis
Nephronex
nephropathy
diabetic n.
reflux n.
nephrosclerosis
malignant n.

nephrosis
congenital n.
nephrostomy
percutaneous n.
nephrotic syndrome
nephrotoxicity
nepiology
Neptazane
nerve
n. block
facial n.
femoral n.
hemorrhoidal n.
n. injury
obturator n.
n. palsy
parasympathetic n.
pelvic n.
pelvic floor n.
perineal n.
presacral n.
pudendal n.
saphenous n.
sciatic n.
thoracolumbar sympathetic n.
nervi erigentes
Nervine
Nervocaine
nervosa
bulimia n.
nervous system
NET-EN
norethindrone enanthate
neural
n. groove
n. tube
n. tube defect (NTD)
neuralgia
mammary n.
Neuramate
neurectomy
presacral n.
neurenteric canal
neuritis
neuroblastoma
neurodevelopment
neurodevelopmental disability
neuroendocrine system
neuroendocrinology
neurofibroma
neurofibromatosis
neurohypophysis
neuroleptic
neurologic, neurological
n. abnormality
n. complication
n. development
n. disorder
n. examination
n. involvement
neuromodulator
neuropathy
femoral n.
nutritional n.
obstetric n.
porphyric n.
retractor n.
neurophysin I
neurophysin II
neurophysiology
neuroplate
neurosecretion
neurosyphilis
neurotensin
neurotransmitter
n. release
neutralization
neutron
fast n.
n. therapy
neutropenia
neonatal n.
nevus, pl. **nevi**
benign n.
melanocytic n.
spider n.
vulvar n.
newborn
hemorrhagic disease of the n.
physiologic jaundice of the n.
transient tachypnea of the n.
New York Heart Association classification of heart disease
Niac
niacin
niacinamide
nialamide
nicardipine
Nico-400
Nicobid
Nicolar
Nicolas-Favre disease

nicotinamide
nicotine
nicotinic acid
nicotinyl alcohol
nicoumalone
nidation
NIDDM
non-insulin-dependent diabetes mellitus
Niemann-Pick disease
nifedipine
nigricans
nipple
accessory n.
n. discharge
inverted n.
out-of-profile n.
n. retraction
n. shield
n. stimulation test
Nipride
Nisentil
nit
Nitabuch's layer
nitrate
miconazole n.
silver n.
nitrazine test
nitrite
amyl n.
Nitro-Bid
Nitrocap
nitrofurantoin
nitrogen
blood urea n. (BUN)
n. mustard
nitroglycerin
Nitroglyn
nitroimidazole compound
Nitrol
Nitrolingual
Nitronet
Nitrong
nitroprusside
sodium n.
nitrosourea
Nitrospan
Nitrostat
nitrous oxide
Nix Cream Rinse
Nizoral
NK cells
natural killer cells
NMR
nuclear magnetic resonance
Noctec
node
aortic n.
axillary lymph n.
Cloquet's n.
femoral lymph n.
gluteal lymph n.
hypogastric lymph n.
iliac n.
inguinal lymph n.
intramammary lymph n.
lymph n.
para-aortic n.
parauterine lymph n.
pelvic lymph n.
periaortic lymph n.
pericervical n.
rectal n.
retroperitoneal n.
sacral lymph n.
subaortic lymph n.'s
ureteral n.
vulvar lymph n.
nodular melanoma
nodule
Hoboken's n.'s
placental site n.
thyroid n.
nomenclature
FIGO n.
nomogram
body mass index n.
nonalkylating agent
non-A, non-B hepatitis
non-breast-feeding woman
noncalcified nodular mass
noncarbonic acid
nonclassic 21-hydroxylase deficiency
noncommunicating uterine horn
nondeciduous placenta
nondisjunction
nonestrogen drug
nonfenestrated forceps
nongranulomatous salpingitis
nonhemolytic aerobic organism
non-Hodgkin's lymphoma
nonimmune
n. fetal hydrops
non-insulin-dependent diabetes mellitus (NIDDM)

noninvasive management
nonketotic hyperglycinemia
nonlactating breast
non-obstetrical claim
nonovulational menstruation
nonoxynol-9
nonoxynol-9/octoxynol-9
nonpalpable abnormality
nonparous
nonradioactive immunoassay
nonreactive immunoassay
non-sex hormone-binding globulin bound testosterone
nonspecific
n. immunotherapy
n. mesenchyme
n. urethritis
n. vaginitis
nonsteroidal anti-inflammatory drug (NSAID)
nonstressed fetus
nonstress test
nonviable
nonvolatile acid
Noonan's syndrome
noradrenaline
Noradryl
Norcept-E 1/35
Nordryl
norepinephrine
norethindrone
n. acetate
n. enanthate (NET-EN)
Norethin 1/35E
Norethin 1/35M
norethisterone
norethynodrel
Norflex
norfloxacin
norgestrel
norgestrel/ethinyl estradiol combination
Norinyl 1 + 35
Norinyl 1 + 50
Norisodrine
Norlestrin 1/50
Norlestrin 2.5/50
Norlutin
normal
n. blood loss
n. midcycle spinnbarkeit
n. ovariotomy
n. pregnancy
n. saline
n. transformation zone
Nor-Mil
Normodyne
normotensive woman
Noroxin
Norpace
Norpanth
Norplant
Norpramin
Nor-Q.D.
19-nortestosterone
19-n. derivative
Norton's operation
nortriptyline
Nortussin
nosocomial infection
note
operative n.
notochord
Novafed
Novantrone
Nova Rectal
novobiocin
Novobutamide
Novochlorhydrate
Novodimenate
Novo-Flurazine
Novofuran
Novo-Hydrazide
Novomepro
Novonidazol
Novopen
Novopen-VK
Novopoxide
Novopramine
Novopropamide
Novo-Ridazine
Novorythro
Novosecobarb
Novosoxazole
Novotetra
Novotriptyn
Nozinan
NSABP
National Surgical Adjuvant Breast Project
NSAID
nonsteroidal anti-inflammatory drug
NTD
neural tube defect
Nubain

nuchal
n. arm
n. cord
Nuck's
N. canal
N. hydrocele
nuclear
n. antigen
n. magnetic resonance (NMR)
n. radiation
nucleic acid probe
nucleosome
nucleotide
nucleus
arcuate n.
steroid n.
nude mouse
null hypothesis
nulligravida
nullipara
nulliparity
nulliparous
number
ovulation n.
Reynolds n.
Numorphan
nutrient requirement
nutrition
fetal n.
maternal n.
parenteral n.
total parenteral n. (TPN)
nutritional
n. neuropathy
n. problem
n. surveillance
Nydrazid
nylidrin hydrochloride
nylon suture material
nympha, pl. **nymphae**
nymphectomy
nymphitis
nymphoncus
nymphotomy
Nyquist frequency
nystatin
Nytilax

O

OA
occiput anterior
OB
obstetrics
Obalan
Obephen
obesity
android o.
o. in endometrial sarcoma
experimental o.
gynecoid o.
Obeval
Obezine
OB/GYN
obstetrics and gynecology
oblique
o. diameter
o. lie
obliquity
Litzmann's o.
Nägele o.
observation
observer variation
obstetric, obstetrical
o. anesthesia
o. conjugate
o. conjugate of the outlet
o. history
o. neuropathy
o. position
obstetrician
high-tech o.
obstetrician-gynecologist
Obstetrics
International Federation of Gynecology and O. (FIGO)
obstetrics (OB)
defensive o.
obstetrics and gynecology (OB/GYN)
obstruction
bowel o.
colonic o.
distal tubal o.
fimbrial o.
gastrointestinal o.
intestinal o.
tubal o.
ureteral o.
urinary tract o.
obstructive
o. dysmenorrhea
o. uropathy
obturator
o. artery
o. fascia
o. nerve
OC-125
occipitoanterior position
occipitofrontal diameter
occipitomental diameter
occipitoposterior position
occipitotransverse position
occiput
o. anterior (OA)
o. posterior (OP)
o. presentation
o. transverse (OT)
occlusion
distal o.
proximal o.
occult
o. blood
o. cancer
occupational history
Ochsner forceps
OCT
oxytocin challenge test
Octamide
Octoxynol-9
ocular
o. involvement
o. manifestation
o. prophylaxis
Ocu-Sol
od gene
Oestrilin
office cystometrics
Ogino-Knaus rule
17-OHP
17-hydroxyprogesterone
oil
camphorated o.
o. cyst
ethiodized o.
mineral o.
ointment
zinc oxide o.

Okazaki fragment
17β-ol-dehydrogenase
oleandomycin phosphate
oligoamnios
oligoasthenospermia
oligogalactia
oligohydramnios
oligomenorrhea
oligospermia
oligozoospermia
oliguria
omentectomy
omentum
lymphocyst o.
OMI
oocyte maturation inhibitor
Omnipen
omphaloangiopagous twins
omphaloangiopagus
omphalocele
omphalorrhagia
omphalorrhea
omphalorrhexis
omphalotomy
omphalotripsy
oncofetal antigen
oncogene
oncogenic
o. agent
o. potential
Oncologists
Society of Gynecologic O.
Oncology
Society of Gynecologic O. (SGO)
oncology
gynecological o.
Oncovin
one-child sterility
one-horned uterus
one-hour glucose tolerance test
one-tail test
oocyesis
oocyte
o. cryopreservation
o. culture
o. donation
o. extrusion
o. maturation inhibitor (OMI)
o. meiosis
primary o.
o. retrieval
oogenesis
oogonium, pl. **oogonia**
oophoralgia
oophorectomy
prophylactic o.
oophoritic cyst
oophoritis
autoimmune o.
oophorocystectomy
oophorocystosis
oophorohysterectomy
oophoroma
oophoropathy
oophoropeliopexy
oophoropexy
oophoroplasty
oophororrhaphy
oophorosalpingectomy
oophorosalpingitis
oophorostomy
oophorotomy
oophorrhagia
oozing
venous o.
OP
occiput posterior
opening
urethral o.
vaginal o.
operation
Baldy's o.
Baudelocque's o.
Bozeman's o.
Brunschwig's o.
cesarean o.
Cotte's o.
Doyle's o.
Emmet's o.
Estes o.
Fothergill's o.
Freund's o.
Gigli's o.
Gilliam's o.
Halsted's o.
Heaney's o.
Kelly's o.
Lash's o.
Le Fort o.
Madlener o.
Manchester o.
Manchester-Fothergil o.
Marshall-Marchetti-Krantz o.
McIndoe's o.

morcellation o.
Norton's o.
obstetrical o.
Pomeroy's o.
Porro o.
Récamier's o.
Saenger's o.
Schauta vaginal o.
Schroeder's o.
Schuchardt's o.
second-look o.
Shirodkar o.
Spinelli o.
Sturmdorf's o.
suprapubic urethrovesical suspension o.
suspensory sling o.
TeLinde o.
transsphenoidal o.
Urban's o.
Waters' o.
Webster's o.
Wertheim's o.

operative
o. laparoscopy
o. note
o. site complication

operculum, gen. **operculi**, pl. **opercula**

ophthalmia
gonorrheal o.
o. neonatorum

opiate
endogenous o.

opioid
o. activity
o. addiction
o. peptide
o. receptor
o. receptor antagonist

opioidergic control impairment

opipramol hydrochloride

opium

opposing wall

opsonization

optical density measurement

Opticrom

Optimine

ora

Oradexon

Oragrafin

oral
o. administration
o. cavity
o. conjugated estrogen
o. contraception
o. contraceptive
o. hormone replacement therapy
o. hypoglycemic

orally administered estrogen

Oramide

Orange
Agent O.

Orap

Orbenin

orciprenaline sulfate

order
admission o.
high fetal o.
preoperative o.'s

Oretic

organ
internal generative o.
nongenital pelvic o.
o. of Rosenmüller
sensory o.
o. transplant
o. transplantation

organism
Gram-negative o.
nonhemolytic aerobic o.

organogenesis

orgasm

orgasmic plateau

origin
histoimmunological o.
parental o.

Orimune

Orinase

oris

ornithine decarboxylase

orphenadrine

Ortho-Creme

Ortho-Gynol

Ortho-Novum 1/35

Ortho-Novum 1/50

Ortho-Novum 7/7/7

Ortho-Novum 10/11

orthopaedic, orthopedic
o. anomaly
o. condition

orthostatic
o. hypotension
o. proteinuria

orthovoltage

Orthoxine
os, gen. **oris**, pl. **ora**
cervical o.
external o.
internal o.
Scanzoni's second o.
Osmoglyn
osmolality
ossa
ossis
osteitis pubis
osteoblast
osteoblast-like cell
osteochondritis
osteocystoma
osteogenesis imperfecta
osteomalacia
osteomyelitis
o. pubis
osteopenia
relative o.
osteoporosis
postmenopausal o.
osteoporotic fracture
osteosarcoma
ostium secundum
O'Sullivan-O'Connor retractor
OT
occiput transverse
otocyst
ouabain
outcome
adverse o.
fetal o.
maternal o.
neonatal o.
obstetrical o.
perinatal o.
pregnancy o.
teratogenic o.
outlet
pelvic o.
vaginal o.
vulvovaginal o.
outline
fetal o.
out-of-phase endometrial biopsy
out-of-profile nipple
outpatient biopsy
output
cardiac o.
urine o.
ovarialgia
ovarian
o. abnormality
o. abscess
o. activity
o. amenorrhea
o. antibody
o. artery
o. cancer
o. carcinoid tumor
o. carcinoma
o. cautery
o. colic
o. cycle
o. cyst
o. cystadenocarcinoma
o. cystadenoma
o. cystectomy
o. cystic teratoma
o. disorder
o. dysgenesis
o. dysgerminoma
o. dysmenorrhea
o. embryonal teratoma
o. endometrioid carcinoma
o. endometriosis
o. estrogen synthesis
o. factor
o. failure
o. fibroma
o. follicle exhaustion
o. fossa
o. function
o. gametogenesis
o. germinal epithelium
o. gonadoblastoma
o. granulosa cell proliferation
o. hormone
o. hyperandrogenism
o. hyperstimulation
o. leiomyoma
o. ligament
o. lymphoma
o. mass
o. metastasis
o. neoplasm
o. plexus
o. pregnancy
o. remnant syndrome
o. response
o. serous tumor
o. steroid
o. steroidogenesis

o. stroma
o. teratoma
o. thecoma
o. torsion
o. tubular adenoma
o. tumor
o. varicocele
o. vein
o. wedge resection
ovariectomy
ovarioabdominal pregnancy
ovariocele
ovariocentesis
ovariocyesis
ovariodysneuria
ovariogenic
ovariohysterectomy
ovariolytic
ovarioncus
ovariopathy
ovariorrhexis
ovariosalpingectomy
ovariosalpingitis
ovariosteresis
ovariostomy
ovariotomy
normal o.
ovaritis
ovarium, pl. **ovaria**
o. bipartitum
o. disjunctum
o. gyratum
o. lobatum
ovary
accessory o.
insensitive o.
mulberry o.
multifollicular o.
palpable postmenopausal o.
polycystic o.
resistant o.
sclerocystic o.
Stein-Leventhal type of polycystic o.
strumal carcinoid of o.
supernumerary o.
transposition of o.
Ovcon
overdistention syndrome
overflow incontinence
overriding
o. aorta
overshoot
over-the-counter medication
overt insulin-dependent diabetes mellitus
oviduct
ampulla of o.
angiomyoma of o.
ovine
o. trophoblast protein-1
ovoid
Manchester o.
ovotestis, pl. **ovotestes**
Ovrette
ovular transmigration
ovulation
o. age
contralateral o.
incessant o.
o. induction
o. number
paracyclic o.
o. rate
spontaneous o.
o. stimulation
ovulational sclerosis
ovulatory
o. age
o. cycle
o. defect
o. disturbance
ovulocyclic
o. porphyria
ovum, pl. **ova**
blighted o.
o. capture
fertilized o.
hamster o.
o. maturation
trapped o.
ovum-capture inhibitor
oxacillin
oxazepam
Oxford Family Planning Association Contraceptive Study
oxidase
diamine o.
monoamine o. (MOA)
oxide
nitrous o.
zinc o.
oximetry
pulse o.
reflectance pulse o.
Ox-Pam

oxprenolol
oxtriphylline
oxybutynin chloride
oxycodone
Oxydess II
oxygen
o. consumption
o. delivery
o. dissociation curve
hyperbaric o.
partial pressure of o.
o. saturation
o. tension
o. toxicity
oxygenated fetal blood
oxygenation
extracorporeal membrane o.
fetal o.
fetal scalp o.
oxygen-diffusing capacity
oxymorphone
oxyphenbutazone
oxyphencyclimine
oxyphenonium bromide
oxytetracycline
oxytocia
oxytocic
o. stimulation
oxytocin
o. analogue
o. augmentation
o. challenge test (OCT)
o. stimulation of labor
oxytocinase

P

^{32}P
phosphorus-32
PA
plasminogen activator
pacemaker
artificial p.
pachysalpingitis
pachysalpingo-ovaritis
pachytene stage
pachyvaginitis
p. cystica
packed
p. cells
packing
pagetic
pagetoid
Paget's disease
pagophagia
Pain
International Association for the Study of P.
pain
abdominal p.
acyclic pelvic p.
after-p.'s
bearing-down p.
bone p.
breast p.
calf p.
epigastric p.
expulsive p.'s
false p.'s
flank p.
hypogastric p.
intermenstrual p.
labor p.'s
low-back p.
lower abdominal p.
middle p.
pelvic p.
periumbilical p.
pleuritic p.
psychogenic pelvic p.
referred pelvic p.
p. relief
shoulder p.
splanchnic pelvic p.
suprapubic p.
painless vaginal bleeding
Pajot's maneuver
palate
cleft p.
palliative surgery
palmar erythema
palmatae
plicae p.
palm leaf pattern
palpable postmenopausal ovary
palpation
palsy
Bell's p.
brachial birth p.
cerebral p.
Erb's p.
facial nerve p.
Klumpke's p.
nerve p.
obstetrical brachial plexus p.
PAMBA
para-aminomethylbenzoic acid
Pamelor
Pamine
pamoate
pampiniform plexus
pancreas
pancreatic pseudocyst
pancreatitis
gallstone p.
Panectyl
Panex
Panmycin
pantothenate
calcium p.
pantothenic acid
Panwarfin
PAPase
phosphatidic acid phosphohydrolase
papaverine
papilla, pl. **papillae**
columnar epithelium p.
papillary
p. adenocarcinoma
p. carcinoma
p. cystadenocarcinoma
p. hidradenoma
papilloma
duct p.
intraductal p.

papillomatosis
juvenile p.
laryngeal p.
subareolar duct p.
Papillomavirus
P. hybridization
P. infection
type 16 *P.*
P. wart
Pap-Kaps
Pap smear
papular
p. dermatitis of pregnancy
papule
pruritic urticarial p.
urticarial p.
papulosis
bowenoid p.
para, para I, para II
para-aminomethylbenzoic acid (PAMBA)
para-aminosalicylic acid
para-aortic
p.-a. irradiation
p.-a. node
p.-a. positivity
p.-a. radiation therapy
paracentesis
paracentric inversion
paracervical
p. anesthesia
p. block
p. injection
p. lymphatics
paracetamol
paracolpitis
paracrine
p. communication
paracyclic ovulation
paracyesis
Paradione
paradoxical incontinence
Paraflex
ParaGard T380A intrauterine copper contraceptive
para I
para II
parakeratosis
multinucleation p.
paralysis, pl. **paralyses**
antigenic p.
Duchenne's p.
facial p.
facial nerve p.
immunologic p.
Klumpke's p.
obstetrical p.
respiratory p.
paralytic ileus
paramedian incision
paramenia
paramesonephric duct
paramethadione
parametrectomy
radical p.
parametrial phlegmon
parametric abscess
parametritic
p. abscess
parametritis
parametrium
paraplegia
congenital spastic p.
infantile spastic p.
parasalpingitis
parasite
intestinal p.
parasitic
p. leiomyoma
p. myoma
parasympathetic
p. nerve
p. nervous system
parathyroid
p. adenoma
p. disease
p. disorder
p. gland
p. hormone
paratubal cyst
paraurethral
p. duct
p. gland
parauterine lymph node
paravaginal
p. hysterectomy
p. soft tissue
paravaginitis
paregoric
parenchyma
parenchymatous mastitis
parentage
parental origin
parenteral
p. alimentation

p. hyperalimentation
p. nutrition
pargyline
Paris method for radium therapy
parity
Parkinson's disease
Parlodel
Parnate
parodynia
paromomycin sulfate
paroophoritic cyst
paroophoritis
paroöphoron
parotid enlargement
parous
parovarian, paraovarian
p. cyst
p. tumor
parovariotomy
parovaritis
parovarium
paroxysmal nocturnal hemoglobinuria
Parsidol
pars tuberalis
part
presenting p.
partial
p. hydatidiform mole
p. pressure of oxygen
p. thromboplastin time (PTT)
particle
alpha p.
particulate
p. matter
p. radiation
partner
sexual p.
parturient
p. canal
parturifacient
parturiometer
parturition
Parvovirus
P. B19
passage
transplacental p.
passive
p. immunity
Pasteur Institute bacillus Calmette-Guérin vaccine
Patau's syndrome
patch
blood p.
moth p.
transdermal medication p.
patency
probe p.
patent ductus arteriosus
paternal age
paternity
Pathilon
Pathocil
pathogen
pathogenesis
pathologic, pathological
p. amenorrhea
p. finding
p. retraction ring
p. rigidity
Pathologists
Cancer Committee of College of American P.
Pathology
International Society for Gynecologic P. (ISGYP)
Society for Gynecologic P.
pathology
hilar cell p.
perinatal p.
uterine p.
pathophysiology
patient
amenorrheic p.
anovulatory p.
antenatal p.
p. education
gynecologic cancer p.
high-risk p.
infertile p.
pregnant cardiac p.
p. response
thalassemic p.
pattern
atypical vessel colposcopic p.
banding p.
chromosomal p.
dysfunctional labor p.
fetal heart rate p.
inactivation p.
mosaic p.
palm leaf p.
prominent ductal p.

pattern *(continued)*
silent fetal heart rate p.
snowflake p.
Pavabid
Pavacap
Pavacen
Pavarine
Pavatest
PCC
postcoital contraception
11p13 chromosome deletion
P_{CO_2}
PCOS
polycystic ovary syndrome
PCR
polymerase chain reaction
PCWP
pulmonary capillary wedge pressure
Peacock's bromide
peak
Bragg p.
Péan forceps
Pearl index
peau d'orange
pectoralis major muscle
Pedersen's speculum
pediatric
p. cocktail
p. gynecology
p. ovarian teratoma
p. vaginoscopy
pedicle clamp
pedicterus
pediculosis pubis
pedigree chart
Pedric
Peganone
pelvic
p. abscess
p. architecture
p. arteriogram
p. artery
p. axis
p. bleeding
p. boost radiotherapy
p. cellulitis
p. congestion syndrome
p. contraction
p. diaphragm
p. discomfort
p. examination
p. exenteration
p. exercise
p. exostosis
p. floor
p. forceps
p. fracture
p. inclination
p. index
p. infection
p. inflammation
p. inflammatory disease (PID)
p. inlet
p. irradiation
p. joint
p. kidney
p. lymphadenectomy
p. lymph node
p. mass
p. nerve
p. node dissection
p. outlet
p. pain
p. peritonitis
p. plane of greatest dimensions
p. plane of inlet
p. plane of least dimensions
p. plane of outlet
p. plexus
p. pole
p. presentation
p. relaxation
p. score
p. support disorder
p. tenderness
p. vein
p. version
pelvic direction
pelvicephalography
pelvicephalometry
pelvic-floor surgery
pelvifixation
pelvigraph
pelvimeter
pelvimetry
computed tomographic p.
CT p.
manual p.
planographic p.
stereoscopic p.
x-ray p.
pelvioperitonitis

pelvioplasty
pelvioscopy, pelvoscopy
pelviotomy
pelviperitonitis
pelvis, pl. **pelves**
android p.
anthropoid p.
contracted p.
cordate p., cordiform p.
Deventer's p.
dwarf p.
flat p.
funnel-shaped p.
gynecoid p.
heart-shaped p.
inverted p.
p. justo major
p. justo minor
juvenile p.
kyphotic p.
longitudinal oval p.
masculine p.
mesatipellic p.
p. nana
p. plana
platypellic p.
platypelloid p.
reniform p.
Robert's p.
round p.
transverse oval p.
pelviscope
pelvitherm
pelvocephalography
Pen A/N
Penbritin
pendulous abdomen
penetrance
penetration
penicillamine
penicillin
p. G
p. G procaine
p. phenoxymethyl
procaine p.
p. V
penile urethra
penis
hypoplastic p.
Pennington clamp
Penrose drain
pentaerythritol tetranitrate
pentamidine isethionate
Pentazine
pentazocine
Penthrane
Pentids
Pentids-P AS
pentobarbital
pentobarbitone
Pentothal
pentoxifylline
Pentritol
penumbra
PenVee K
PEP
progestogen-dependent endometrial protein
peptic
p. ulcer
peptide
amino-terminal p.
atrial natriuretic p.
brain p.
corticotropin-like intermediate lobe p.
endogenous opioid p.
gonadotropin-releasing p.
gonadotropin releasing hormone-associated p. (GAP)
gonadotropin-releasing hormone-like p.
opioid p.
vasoactive intestinal p. (VIP)
Peptococcus
Peptostreptococcus
Percocet
Percodan
percussion
abdominal p.
percutaneous
p. blood sampling
p. drainage
p. fetal transfusion
p. nephrostomy
p. nephrostomy catheter
p. umbilical blood sampling (PUBS)
Perduretas Anfetamina
Pereyra procedure
perforation
ileal p.
uterine p.

performance
reproductive p.
perfusion
placental p.
renal p.
uteroplacental p.
pergolide
Pergonal
Periactin
periaortic lymph node
periappendicitis
p. decidualis
periarteritis nodosa
pericanalicular fibroadenoma
pericentric inversion
pericervical node
pericolpitis
periconceptional rubella
peridural
p. analgesia
p. anesthesia
perihepatitis
perilobular connective tissue
perimenopausal woman
perimenopause
perimesonephric
p. cyst
p. vaginal cyst
perimetritic
perimetritis
perinatal
p. acidosis
p. asphyxia
p. death
p. distress
p. effect
p. medicine
p. morbidity
p. mortality
p. mortality rate
p. outcome
p. pathology
p. risk factor
p. transmission
perinate
perinatologist
perinatology
perineal
p. analgesia
p. anesthesia
p. body
p. defect
p. disruption
p. hygiene
p. nerve
p. scar
p. sphincter disruption
perineorrhaphy
vaginal p.
perineotomy
perineovaginal fistula
perinephric
p. abscess
p. phlegmon
perineum
period
canalicular p.
effective refractory p.
embryonic p.
fertile p.
intrapartum p.
last menstrual p. (LMP)
menstrual p.
missed p.
postpartum p.
previous menstrual p. (PMP)
pseudoglandular p.
puerperal p.
saccular p.
safe p.
terminal saccular p.
periodic
p. auscultation
p. patient assessment
periodicity
perioophoritis
perioophorosalpingitis
periostitis
pubic symphysis p.
periovaritis
peripartum cardiomyopathy
peripheral
p. androgen activity
p. hormone level
p. mononeuropathy
p. placental separation
p. vascular shock
periportal hemorrhagic necrosis
perirectal fascia
perisalpingitis
perisalpingo-ovaritis
peristalsis
intestinal p.
peritomy

peritoneal
p. catheter
p. cavity fluid
p. cytology
p. dialysis
p. fluid
p. implant
p. lavage
p. suturing
peritoneum
visceral p.
peritonitis
meconium p.
pelvic p.
Peritrate
peritubal adhesion
periumbilical pain
periurethral
p. gland
p. structure
perivaginitis
periventricular leukomalacia
Perlutal
permethrin
Permitil
pernicious
p. anemia
peroxide
hydrogen p.
zinc p.
perphenazine
Persantine
persistence
persistent
p. anovulation
p. estrogen secretion
p. fetal circulation
p. ovarian mass
p. trophoblastic tumor
personal injury law
Pertofrane
per vias naturales
pessary
cube type p.
diaphragm p.
donut p.
Dumontpallier's p.
Gariel's p.
Hodge's p.
Mayer's p.
Menge's p.
prostaglandin p.
ring p.
Smith-Hodge p.
pethidine
Peutz-Jeghers syndrome
Pfannenstiel's incision
P-fimbriae
Pfizerpen
P. AS
Pflüger
cord of P.
PG
prostaglandin
PGE_2-gel cervical priming
PGG
prostaglandin G
PGH
prostaglandin H
PGI_2
prostacyclin
PGSI
prostaglandin synthetase inhibitor
pH
fetal blood pH
vaginal pH
phagocytosis
phallus
Phaneuf uterine artery forceps
phantom
p. pregnancy
Schultze's p.
Pharmaceutical
Wells v. Ortho P.
pharmacokinetics
quinolone p.
pharyngeal gonococcal infection
phase
active p.
catagen p.
fertile p.
follicular p.
hair growth p.
hyperprolactinemia-associated luteal p.
implantation p.
inadequate luteal p.
latent p.
luteal p.
mitosis p. (M phase)
proliferative p.
secretory p.
telogen p.
phenacetin

phenanthrene
Phenaphen
Phenazine
Phenazo
phenazocine
Phenazodine
phenazone
phenazopyridine
phencyclidine
phendimetrazine
phenelzine
Phenergan
Phenetron
phenindione
pheniramine
phenobarbital
phenobarbitone
phenolsulfonphthalein (PSP)
  p. test
phenomenon, pl. **phenomena**
  all or none p.
  Arias-Stella p.
  memory p.
  piezoelectric p.
  rebound p.
  recall p.
  Strassman's p.
phenothiazine
phenotype
phenotypic sex
phenoxybenzamine hydrochloride
phenoxymethyl
  penicillin p.
phenoxymethylpenicillin
phenprocoumon
phensuximide
phentanyl
phentermine
phentolamine
phenylalanine
  p. hydroxylase
L-phenylalanine mustard
phenylbutazone
phenylephrine
phenylhydantoin
phenylketonuria (PKU)
  maternal p.
  preconceptionally treated p.
phenylpropanolamine
phenyltoloxamine
phenytoin
pheochromocytoma
Pheryl E
Philadelphia chromosome
phimosis, pl. **phimoses**
  p. vaginalis
phlebitis
  puerperal p.
  suppurative p.
phlebography
phlebometritis
phlebothrombosis
phlegmasia
  p. alba dolens
  cellulitic p.
  p. dolens
  thrombotic p.
phlegmon
  parametrial p.
  perinephric p.
phlegmonous mastitis
phonocardiography
phosphatase
  acid p.
  alkaline p.
  lysosomal acid p.
phosphate
  chromic p.
phosphatidic acid phosphohydrolase (PAPase)
phosphatidylcholine
  disaturated p.
phosphatidylglycerol
phosphohydrolase
  phosphatidic acid p. (PAPase)
Phospholine Iodide
phospholipase
  p. A_2
  p. activity
  p. C
  p. C-protein kinase C pathway
phospholipid
  p. antibody
phosphorus
phosphorus-32 (^{32}P)
phosphorylation
  myosin light-chain p.
photocoagulation
  laser p.
photodynamic therapy
photomicrograph
photon
photostethoscope
phototherapy

photovaporization
laser p.
phthalylsulfacetamide
phthalylsulfathiazole
phygogalactic
phylloquinone
physical examination
physician-applied force
physician's responsibility
physiologic, physiological
p. amenorrhea
p. childbirth
p. follicular regulation
p. icterus
p. jaundice
p. replacement dose
p. retraction ring
p. sclerosis
p. third-stage management
physiologist
fetal p.
physiology
maternal p.
physometra
physopyosalpinx
physostigmine
phytoagglutinin
phytomenadione
phytonadione
pica
pick-up
Adson p.-u.'s
rat tooth p.-u.'s
PID
pelvic inflammatory disease
Pierre Robin syndrome
piezoelectric phenomenon
PIF
prolactin inhibiting factor
pigmentation
pigmented lesion
pileus
pill
birth control p.
combined birth control p.
morning-after p.
Pilocar
pilocarpine
Piloptic
pilosebaceous unit
Pima
pimozide
Pinard's maneuver
pindolol
pineal gland
pinworm
p. vaginitis
pion
PIOPED
Prospective Investigation of Pulmonary Embolus Diagnosis
Pipelle endometrial suction curette
piperacetazine
piperacillin
piperazine
p. dione
p. estrone sulfate
piperidolate hydrochloride
Piper's forceps
Pipracil
Pitocin
Pitressin
pituitary
p. adenoma
p. axis
p. cell
p. desensitization
p. disease
p. disorder
p. gland
p. gland function
p. gland transplantation
p. gland tumor
p. gonadotropin
p. hormone
p. necrosis
p. response
pituitary-ovarian function
pivot lock
PK
pyruvate kinase
PKU
phenylketonuria
place
birth p.
placenta
accessory p.
p. accreta
p. accreta vera
adherent p.
annular p.
battledore p.
bidiscoidal p.
p. biloba
p. bipartita

placenta *(continued)*
central p. previa
chorioallantoic p.
chorioamnionic p.
p. circumvallata
cotyledonary p.
deciduate p.
dichorionic p.
dichorionic diamniotic p.
p. diffusa
p. dimidiata
disperse p.
p. duplex
endotheliochorial p.
endothelio-endothelial p.
epitheliochorial p.
p. extrachorales
p. fenestrata
hemochorial p.
horseshoe p.
incarcerated p.
p. increta
labyrinthine p.
p. marginata
p. membranacea
monochorionic diamniotic p.
monochorionic monoamniotic p.
p. multiloba
nondeciduous p.
p. panduraformis
p. percreta
p. previa
p. previa centralis
p. previa creta
p. previa marginalis
p. previa partialis
p. reflexa
p. reniformis
retained p.
Schultze's p.
p. spuria
succenturiate p.
supernumerary p.
total p. previa
p. triloba
p. tripartita
p. triplex
twin p.
p. velamentosa
villous p.
zonary p.

placental
p. abruption
p. aromatase deficiency
p. barrier
p. bleeding site
p. cotyledon
p. dysfunction syndrome
p. dystocia
p. extrusion
p. fragment
p. giant cell
p. grade
p. grading
p. growth
p. hemorrhage
p. hormone
p. immunology
p. implantation
p. infarct
p. insufficiency
p. insulinase
p. lactogen
p. leakage
p. localization
p. membrane
p. metastasis
p. migration
p. perfusion
p. polyp
p. presentation
p. protein
p. secretion
p. separation
p. septum
p. sign
p. site
p. site nodule
p. souffle
p. stage
p. steroid
p. sulfatase deficiency
p. thickness
p. thrombosis
p. tissue
p. transfer
p. transfusion
p. villus
p. weight

placental-site gestational trophoblastic disease

placentascan

placentation
hemochorioendothelial p.

placentitis
placentography
indirect p.
placentoma
Placidyl
plague vaccine
Plan
Health Insurance P. (HIP)
plane
first parallel pelvic p.
fourth parallel pelvic p.
p. of midpelvis
p. of pelvic canal
pelvic p. of greatest dimensions
pelvic p. of inlet
pelvic p. of least dimensions
pelvic p. of outlet
second parallel pelvic p.
third parallel pelvic p.
wide p.
planning
family p.
planographic pelvimetry
plant alkaloid
planus
lichen p.
plasma
p. albumin
p. cell balanitis
p. cell mastitis
p. fraction
fresh frozen p. (FFP)
frozen p.
p. iron-binding capacity
p. iron concentration
p. level
p. protein
p. volume
plasmapheresis
plasmin
plasminogen
p. activator (PA)
plastic cup vacuum extractor
plate
basal p.
vaginal p.
plateau
orgasmic p.
platelet
p. adhesion
p. aggregation
p. antigen
p. concentrate
p. count
p. disorder
p. function test
low p.'s
maternal p.
p. neutralization procedure
p. transfusion
platelet-activating factor
platelet-associated antibody
platelet-derived growth factor
platinum
platypellic
p. pelvis
platypelloid
p. pelvis
Plegine
pleomastia, pleomazia
plethysmography
impedance p.
pleural effusion
pleuritic pain
pleurodesis
tetracycline p.
plexus
Auerbach's p.
brachial p.
cavernous p.
Frankenhäuser's p.
hypogastric p.
ovarian p.
pampiniform p.
pelvic p.
submucosal p.
superior mesenteric p.
vaginal venous p.
plica, pl. **plicae**
plicamycin
ploidy
plug
p. flow
meconium p.
mucous p.
silicone p.
plural pregnancy
PMP
previous menstrual period
PMS
premenstrual syndrome
pneumatic compression
pneumatosis cystoides intestinalis
pneumococcal vaccine

pneumocystiasis
***Pneumocystis carinii* pneumonia**
pneumocystography
pneumocystosis
pneumohydrometra
pneumonia
acute interstitial p.
p. alba of Virchow
chickenpox p.
congenital p.
interstitial plasma cell p.
intrauterine p.
Pneumocystis carinii p.
varicella p.
pneumonitis
aspiration p.
chemical p.
viral p.
pneumonocyte
type II p.
pneumoperitoneum
pneumosalpingography
Pneumovax 23
Pnu-Imune 23
pocket
amniotic fluid p.
podalic
p. extraction
p. version
podofilox
podophyllin
point
p. A
p. B
cardinal p.'s
p. mutation
trigger p.
poisoning
carbon monoxide p.
pokeweed mitogen (PWM)
polar
p. body
p. presentation
Polaramine
polarization
fluorescent p.
pole
cephalic p.
pelvic p.
poliomyelitis
polyamine
polyarteritis nodosa
polybutester
polychlorinated biphenyl
Polycillin
polyclonal antibody
polycyesis
polycystic
p. fibrous dysplasia
p. kidney disease
p. ovary
p. ovary syndrome (PCOS)
p. renal disease
polycythemia
p. vera
polydactylism
polydimethylsiloxane
polydioxanone
polyembryony
polyester suture material
polyethylene suture material
polygalactia
polygalactide suture
polygenic
p. disorder
p. inheritance
polyglandular syndrome
polyglycol suture
polyglyconate suture
polyhydramnios
polyhypermenorrhea
polyhypomenorrhea
polymastia, polymazia
polymenorrhea
polymerase chain reaction (PCR)
polymicrobial bacteremia
polymorphic eruption of pregnancy
polymorphism
restriction fragment length p. (RFLP)
Polymox
polymyositis
primary idiopathic p.
polymyxin
p. B sulfate
polyneuritis
polyostotic fibrous dysplasia
polyp
adenomatous p.
cervical p.
endocervical p.
endometrial p.
fibrinous p.
placental p.
polypectomy
polyploidy

polypoid hyperplasia
polypropylene
p. fascial strip
p. suture material
polysomy
sex chromosomal p.
polythelia
polythiazide
polyvalent
p. pneumococcal vaccine
Pomeroy's operation
ponderal index
Pondimin
Pontocaine
pool
vaginal p.
popcorn-like calcification
porphyria
acute intermittent p.
intermittent p.
ovulocyclic p.
porphyric neuropathy
porphyrin metabolism disorder
Porro
P. hysterectomy
P. operation
portal hypertension
Porter-Silber reaction
portio vaginalis
Portland
hemoglobin P.
position
dorsal birthing p.
English p.
fetal p.
fetal head p.
frontoanterior p.
frontoposterior p.
frontotransverse p.
genucubital p.
genupectoral p.
knee-chest p.
knee-elbow p.
lateral recumbent p.
left frontoanterior p. (LFA)
left frontoposterior p. (LFP)
left frontotransverse p. (LFT)
left mentoanterior p. (LMA)
left mentoposterior p. (LMP)
left mentotransverse p. (LMT)
left occipitoanterior p. (LOA)
left occipitoposterior p. (LOP)
left occipitotransverse p. (LOT)
left sacroanterior p. (LSA)
left sacroposterior p. (LSP)
left sacrotransverse p. (LST)
lithotomy p.
maternal p.
maternal birthing p.
mentoanterior p.
mentoposterior p.
mentotransverse p.
obstetric p.
occipitoanterior p.
occipitoposterior p.
occipitotransverse p.
right acromiodorsoposterior p.
right frontoanterior p. (RFA)
right frontoposterior p. (RFP)
right frontotransverse p. (RFT)
right mentoanterior p. (RMA)
right mentoposterior p. (RMP)
right mentotransverse p. (RMT)
right occipitoanterior p. (ROA)
right occipitoposterior p. (ROP)
right occipitotransverse p. (ROT)
right sacroanterior p. (RSA)
right sacroposterior p. (RSP)
right sacrotransverse p. (RST)
sacroanterior p.
sacroposterior p.
sacrotransverse p.
semiprone p.
Simon's p.
Sims p.
supine p.
Walcher p.

positivity
lymph node p.
para-aortic p.
postadolescence
postaugmentation
postbiopsy
postcoital
p. contraception (PCC)
p. estrogen
p. test
postconception age
postdate
p. pregnancy
postdatism
posterior
p. asynclitism
p. commissure
p. fossa cyst
occiput p. (OP)
p. pelvic exenteration
right occiput p.
p. sagittal diameter
p. urethritis
p. vaginismus
posthetomy
postinflammatory adenopathy
postlumpectomy
postmature
postmaturity
p. syndrome
postmenarchal
p. bleeding
p. cycle
postmenopausal
p. amenorrhea
p. atrophy
p. bleeding
p. body mass
p. bone loss
p. estrogen replacement therapy
p. hirsutism
p. osteoporosis
p. ovary
p. replacement
p. syndrome
postmenopause
postmenstrual stress
postmolar contraception
postmortem
p. delivery
p. study
postnatal
p. year
postoperative
p. bladder dysfunction
p. care
p. chemotherapy
p. complication
p. cystitis
p. fever workup
p. pelvic radiation
p. radiation
p. radiotherapy
p. sepsis
p. seroma
p. shock
p. symptom analysis
p. voiding dysfunction
postpartum
p. amenorrhea
p. blues
p. cardiomyopathy
p. care
p. depression
p. hemolytic uremic syndrome
p. hypertension
p. infection
p. malignant nephrosclerosis
p. period
p. pituitary necrosis syndrome
p. psychosis
p. tetanus
p. thyroiditis
postpill amenorrhea
postpuberal, postpubertal
postpuberty
postpubescent
postradiation
p. cystitis
p. fistula
p. periureteral fibrosis
postreduction
p. mammoplasty
postrubella syndrome
postsurgical fat necrosis
postterm
p. infant
p. pregnancy
posttherapy change
posttraumatic fat necrosis
post-tubal ligation syndrome

postulates
  Koch's p.
postural
  p. deformity
  p. version
posture
  fetal p.
potassium
  p. bromide
  p. chloride
  p. citrate
  p. gluconate
  p. hydroxide
  p. iodide
potential
  oncogenic p.
Potter's
  P. syndrome
  P. version
pouch
  continent urinary p.
  Douglas' p.
  rectouterine p.
Pourcelot index
povidone-iodine
  p.-i. douching
powder pseudocalcification
practitioner
Practitioners
  Royal College of
   General P. (RCGP)
Prader-Willi syndrome
Prague maneuver
pralidoxime chloride
Pratt dilator
prazosin hydrochloride
preadolescent vaginal bleeding
preantral follicle
precancerous lesion
Precef
precipitate
  p. labor
precipitin
precision
preclinical carcinoma
precocious
  p. pseudopuberty
  p. puberty
preconception care
predecidual
prediction
  perinatal distress p.
  prenatal risk p.
  scar p.
predictive
  p. value of negative test
  p. value of positive test
  p. value of test
predictor
  morbidity p.
  mortality p.
prednisolone
prednisone
preeclampsia
  early-onset p.
  p. headache
  superimposed p.
preeclamptic toxemia
pregnancy
  abdominal p.
  aborted ectopic p.
  accidental p.
  p. achievement
  acute fatty liver of p.
  adolescent p.
  ampullar p.
  at-risk p.
  p. belief
  bigeminal p.
  bilateral ectopic p.
  bilateral simultaneous p.'s
  bilateral simultaneous
   tubal p.'s
  broad ligament p.
  p. cell
  cervical p.
  chemical p.
  cholestatic hepatosis of p.
  combined p.
  p. complication
  compound p.
  cornual p.
  p. dating
  ectopic p.
  epulis of p.
  extraamniotic p.
  extrachorial p.
  extramembranous p.
  extrauterine p.
  fallopian p.
  false p.
  fatty liver of p.
  full-term p.
  grand p.
  hepatic p.

pregnancy *(continued)*
heterotopic p.
high-risk p.
p. hormone
hydatid p.
idiopathic cholestasis of p.
interstitial p.
intrahepatic cholestasis of p.
intraligamentary p.
intramural p.
intraperitoneal p.
intrauterine p.
late p.
p. loss
p. luteoma
p. management
mask of p.
mesometric p.
molar p.
multifetal p.
multiple p.
mural p.
near-term p.
p. outcome
ovarian p.
ovarioabdominal p.
pelvic malignancy in p.
pernicious anemia of p.
phantom p.
plural p.
polymorphic light eruption of p.
postdate p.
postterm p.
previous p.
prolonged p.
pruritic urticarial papules and plaques of p.
p. record
recurrent jaundice of p.
refractory anemia of p.
secondary abdominal p.
singleton p.
splenic p.
spurious p.
successful p.
p. test
toxemia of p.
toxemic rash of p.
treatment-associated p.
treatment-independent p.
tubal p.
tuboabdominal p.
tubo-ovarian p.
tubouterine p.
p. tumor
twin p.
unplanned p.
uterine p.
uteroabdominal p.
p. wastage
p. zone protein

pregnancy-associated
p.-a. globulin
p.-a. hypoplastic anemia
p.-a. plasma protein

pregnancy-induced hypertension

pregnancy-specific protein

pregnane

pregnanediol
p. glucuronate

5β-pregnane-3,20-dione

pregnanetriol

pregnant

pregnenolone

preimplantation

preinvasive cervical disease

prelabor

Prelu-2

premalignant
p. disease
p. lesion

premammary abscess

Premarin

premature
p. adrenarche
p. airway closure
p. amnion rupture
p. birth
p. centromere division
p. delivery
p. infant
p. labor
p. luteal regression
p. menopause
p. ovarian failure
p. pubarche
p. rupture of membrane (PROM)
p. thelarche
p. uterine contraction inhibition
p. ventricular contraction (PVC)

prematurity
retinopathy of p.

premenarchal vulvovaginitis
premenopausal
premenstrual
p. edema
p. salivary syndrome
p. syndrome (PMS)
p. tension
premenstruum
prenatal
p. care
p. detection
p. diagnosis
p. diethylstilbestrol exposure
p. genetic diagnosis
p. genetics
p. mortality
p. risk factor
p. risk prediction
p. screening
p. selection
p. sex determination
p. treatment
p. ultrasound
preoperative
p. management
p. orders
p. pulse
p. radiation
p. shaving
p. symptom analysis
preovulatory
p. follicle
p. LH surge
preparation
bowel p.
prepregnancy care
prepuberal, prepubertal
prepubescent
prerenal azotemia
prereproductive
presacral
p. nerve
p. neurectomy
p. sympathectomy
prescription
presentation
acromion p.
breech p.
brow p.
cephalic p.
complete breech p.
compound p.
face p.
footling p., foot p.
frank breech p.
full breech p.
head p.
incomplete breech p.
incomplete foot p.
incomplete knee p.
knee p.
mentoanterior p.
mentoposterior p.
occiput p.
pelvic p.
placental p.
polar p.
shoulder p.
sincipital p.
transverse p.
vertex p.
presenting part
pressor
p. response
pressure
arterial blood p.
blood p.
central venous p. (CVP)
colloid osmotic p. (COP)
continuous positive airway p. (CPAP)
intra-abdominal p.
intravesical p.
maternal abdominal p.
pulmonary capillary wedge p. (PCWP)
p. transmission
urethral p.
preterm
p. birth
p. delivery
p. infant
p. labor
p. labor arrest
p. neonate
prevalence
prevention
prevesical space of Retzius
previa, praevia
previable fetus
previous
p. maternal immunity
p. menstrual period (PMP)
p. pregnancy
previus

PRF
prolactin releasing factor
primaquine
primarily resutured episiotomy
Primatene
primidone
primigravida
elderly p.
priming
cervical p.
primipara
primiparity
primiparous
primitive
p. groove
p. streak
primordial
p. follicle
p. germ cell
primordium
Principen
principle
Doppler p.
Fick p.
Frank-Starling p.
Priscoline
Probalan
proband
Pro-Banthine
probe
endovaginal p.
nucleic acid p.
p. patency
ribonucleic acid p.
transvaginal transducer p.
probenecid
problem
dietary p.
growth p.
intersex p.
nutritional p.
psychosexual p.
procainamide
procaine
p. penicillin
penicillin G p.
Procan SR
procarbazine
Procardia
procedure
admittance p.
Aldridge sling p.
Bricker p.
Burch p.
Chassar moir sling p.
diagnostic p.
dot-blot p.
Estes p.
Everard Williams p.
fascial sling p.
Gepfert p.
Goebell-Stoeckel-Frangenheim p.
interventional p.
intestinal bypass p.
Kelly plication p.
Lash p.
Marshall-Marchetti-Krantz p.
Martius p.
McDonald p.
Meigs-Okabayashi p.
Pereyra p.
platelet neutralization p.
Raz p.
Richter and Albrich p.
Shauta-Aumreich p.
Shirodkar p.
sling p.
Stamey's modification of Pereyra p.
Stanley Way p.
process
freezing p.
immune p.
quality assurance p.
prochlorperazine
procidentia
p. uteri
proctitis
proctocolpoplasty
proctoelytroplasty
proctosigmoiditis
proctosigmoidoscopy
procyclidine
Procytox
product
alpha-1 thymosin p.
blood p.
fibrin degradation p.
prodynorphin
proenkephalin A
proenkephalin B
profenamine
profile
biophysical p.
coagulation p.

lung p.
protein p.
urethral pressure p.
velocity flow p.
Progestasert
progestational
p. agent
p. challenge
p. protection
p. therapy
progesterone
p. breakthrough bleeding
p. challenge test
p. dermatitis
p. metabolism
micronized p.
p. myometrial level
parenteral p.
p. receptor
p. secretion
serum p.
p. synthesis
urinary free p.
p. withdrawal bleeding
progesterone-releasing T-shaped device
progestin
C_{21} p.
p. oral contraceptive
progestin-impregnated vaginal ring
progestins-19-nortestosterone derivative
progestogen
p. support therapy
progestogen-dependent endometrial protein (PEP)
Proglycem
prognosis
clinical p.
prognostic
p. factor
p. indicator
p. scoring system
progression
intraepithelial disease p.
tumor p.
progressive systemic sclerosis
Project
Breast Cancer Detection Demonstration P. (BCDDP)
National Collaborative Diethylstilbestrol Adenosis P. (DESAD)
National Surgical Adjuvant Breast P. (NSABP)
prokaryote
prolactin
p. inhibiting factor (PIF)
plasma p.
p. regulation
p. releasing factor (PRF)
p. secretion
serum p.
p. stimulation
p. suppression
prolactinoma
bromocriptine-resistant p.
estrogen-induced p.
prolactin-secreting
p.-s. adenoma
p.-s. macroadenoma
prolamine
prolan
prolapse
cervical p.
p. of the corpus luteum
first degree p.
mitral valve p.
second degree p.
third degree p.
p. of umbilical cord
urethral p.
uterine p.
p. of the uterus
vaginal p.
vaginal stump p.
vaginal vault p.
proliferation
proliferative phase
proline
Prolixin
Proloid
prolonged
p. gestation
p. labor
p. pregnancy
p. rupture
Proloprim
PROM
premature rupture of membrane
promazine hydrochloride
promethazine
p. hydrochloride

prominence
Rokitansky p.
pronatis
pronephros
Pronestyl
pronuclear stage tubal transfer (PROST)
pronucleus
pro-opiocortin
pro-opiomelanocortin
proopiomelanocortin
pro-oxyphysin
Propaderm
propantheline bromide
prophase
prophylactic
p. antibiotic
p. aspirin use
p. chemotherapy
p. heparin
p. immunization
p. oophorectomy
p. red-cell transfusion
p. tetracycline
prophylaxis
aspiration p.
neonatal ocular p.
ocular p.
silver nitrate eye p.
vitamin K p.
propionicacidemia
propositus
propoxyphene
propranolol
pro-pressophysin
propria
lamina p.
propylthiouracil
Propyl-Thyracil
prorenin
plasma p.
prorenin-renin-angiotensin system
Prospective Investigation of Pulmonary Embolus Diagnosis (PIOPED)
PROST
pronuclear stage tubal transfer
prostacyclin (PGI_2)
prostaglandin (PG)
p. biosynthesis
p. E
p. E_2
p. E_2 gel
p. F_2
p. $F_{2\alpha}$
p. G (PGG)
p. H (PGH)
p. I_2
p. metabolism
p. pessary
p. suppository
p. synthase
p. synthesis inhibition
p. synthesis inhibitor
p. synthetase inhibitor (PGSI)
prostanoid
Prostaphlin
prostatic utricle
prosthesis
valvular p.
Prostigmin
Prostin/15M
protamine
protection
progestational p.
protein
binding p.
p. binding
p. C
carrier p.
C-reactive p.
endometrial p.
follicle regulatory p. (FRP)
G p.
gonadotrophin-releasing hormone-like p.
H-ras p21 p.
myeloma p.
placental p.
plasma p.
pregnancy-associated plasma p.
pregnancy-specific p.
pregnancy zone p.
p. profile
progestogen-dependent endometrial p. (PEP)
p. S
p. standard
thyroxine-binding p. (TBP)
vitamin D-binding p.
protein-1
ovine trophoblast p.
protein kinase C

proteinuria
gestational p.
orthostatic p.
proteolytic enzyme
Proteus
Prothazine
prothrombin time
protocol
modified Bagshawe p. (MBP)
proton
proto-oncogene
c-fms p.-o.
HER-2/neu p.-o.
Protopam
Protostat
protraction
protriptyline
Proval
Proventil
Provera
proximal
p. occlusion
p. tubal blockage
Prozac
Prozine-50
prurigo
p. gestationis
pruritic
p. urticarial papule
pruritus
p. gravidarum
p. vulvae
vulvar p.
psammoma
pseudocalcification
powder p.
pseudocyesis
monosymptomatic delusional p.
pseudocyst
pancreatic p.
pseudodeciduosis
pseudoephedrine hydrochloride
pseudogestational sac
pseudoglandular period
pseudohermaphrodite
pseudohermaphroditism
female p.
male p.
pseudohypoparathyroidism
pseudointraligamentous
pseudolymphoma
pseudomembranous
p. colitis
p. enterocolitis
pseudomenopause
pseudomenstruation
Pseudomonas
P. exotoxin
pseudomosaicism
pseudomyxoma peritonei
pseudopolyp
pseudoprecocious puberty
pseudopregnancy
pseudopuberty
precocious p.
pseudosarcoma
botryoid p.
pseudotoxemia
pseudotumor
p. cerebri
trophoblastic p.
psoriasis
vulvar p.
psoriatic arthritis
PSP
phenolsulfonphthalein
psychiatric
p. disorder
psychoactive drug
psychogenic pelvic pain
psychological
p. effect
p. stress
p. trauma
psychoprophylaxis
psychosexual problem
psychosis, pl. **psychoses**
climacteric p.
gestational p.
involutional p.
postpartum p.
psychosocial
p. adjustment
p. support
psychosomatic disease
psychotherapy
psychotropic drug
Pthirus pubis
PTT
partial thromboplastin time
ptyalism
pubarche
premature p.
puberal, pubertal

pubertas precox
puberty
complete precocious p.
constitutional precocious p.
delayed p.
factitious precocious p.
heterosexual precocious p.
iatrogenic precocious p.
idiopathic precocious p.
incomplete p.
incomplete precocious p.
p. initiation
precocious p.
pseudoprecocious p.
true precocious p.
pubescence
pubescent
pubic
p. arch
p. hair
pubiotomy
pubis
arcuate ligament of p.
mons p.
osteomyelitis p.
symphysis p.
pubococcygeal muscle
puborectal muscle
PUBS
percutaneous umbilical blood sampling
pudendal
p. anesthesia
p. artery
p. block
p. hematocele
p. nerve
pudendum, pl. **pudenda**
puerpera, pl. **puerperae**
puerperal
p. convulsions
p. eclampsia
p. fever
p. hematoma
p. infection
p. mastitis
p. morbidity
p. period
p. phlebitis
p. sepsis
p. septicemia
p. tetanus
puerperant
puerperium, pl. **puerperia**
pulmonary
p. angiography
p. artery catheterization
p. artery/ductus view
p. blood flow
p. capillary wedge pressure (PCWP)
p. diffusing capacity
p. dysmaturity syndrome
p. edema
p. embolism
p. function
p. function tests
p. hypertension
p. hypoplasia
p. infarction
p. injury
p. maturation
p. metastasis
p. resection
p. stenosis
p. thromboembolism
p. tuberculosis
p. vascular bed
pulsatile
p. discharge
p. GnRH administration
p. human menopausal gonadotropin
p. release
pulsatility
p. index
intrinsic p.
pulse
p. frequency
maternal p.
p. oximetry
preoperative p.
pump
breast p.
insulin p.
punch
p. biopsy
p. biopsy forceps
Keyes p.
Keyes dermatologic p.
punctate
pure gonadal dysgenesis
purine
Purinethol

purpura
alloimmune neonatal thrombocytopenic p.
autoimmune thrombocytopenic p.
idiopathic thrombocytopenic p. (ITP)
immune thrombocytopenic p. (ITP)
thrombocytopenic p.
thrombotic thrombocytopenic p. (TTP)
purse-string suture
putrescine
P value
PVC
premature ventricular contraction
P.V. Carpine Liquifilm
PVF K
Pvu II
PWM
pokeweed mitogen
pyelogram
intravenous p.
pyelography
intravenous p. (IVP)
pyelonephritis
p. in exenteration
pyloric stenosis
pyocolpocele
pyocolpos
pyogenic
p. granuloma
p. salpingitis
pyometra
pyometritis
pyomyoma
uterine p.
pyo-ovarium
Pyopen
pyophysometra
pyosalpingitis
pyosalpingo-oophoritis
pyosalpingo-oothecitis
pyosalpinx
pyrantel pamoate
pyrazinamide
pyrexia
maternal p.
Pyribenzamine
Pyridiate
Pyridium
pyridostigmine
pyridoxine
pyrilamine maleate
pyrimethamine
pyrimidine
Pyrinyl
pyrogen
endogenous p.
pyroglutamic acidemia
pyropoikilocytosis
pyrosis
pyruvate
p.
p. decarboxylase
p. kinase (PK)
pyrvinium pamoate
pyuria

Q

Q band
Q-tip test
quadrantectomy
quadruplet
quality assurance
quantitation
amniotic fluid q.
Quarzan
Questran
Quibron
quick
quickening
quiescence
uterine q.
quinacrine hydrochloride
Quinaglute
quinalbarbitone sodium
Quinamm
quinate
quinethazone
quingestanol acetate
Quinidex Extentabs
quinidine
quinine
quinolone
Quinora
quintuplet
Davis q.

R

R
roentgen
^{226}Ra
radium-226
rabies
r. immune globulin
r. vaccine
rad
radial
r. artery
r. scar
r. sclerosing lesion
radiation
r. cystitis
diagnostic r.
r. dose
r. dysplasia
electromagnetic r.
intraoperative r.
ionizing r.
nuclear r.
orthovoltage r.
particulate r.
postoperative r.
postoperative pelvic r.
preoperative r.
state-of-the-art r.
supervoltage r.
r. therapy
tissue tolerance to r.
r. tolerance
whole abdominal r.
radical
r. excision
free hydroxyl r.
r. hysterectomy
r. mastectomy
r. parametrectomy
r. surgery
r. vulvectomy
radioactive
r. colloid
r. gold
r. immunoassay
radiocontrast material
radiocurable
radiofibrinogen uptake scan
radiography
chest r.
digital r.
radioimmunoassay
radioiodine
radioisotope
radiological examination
radiologist-referred diagnostic imaging
radiommunoassay (RIA)
radionuclide
r. venography
radioreceptor assay
radiosensitivity
radiotherapy
abdominal strip r.
adjuvant r.
pelvic boost r.
postoperative r.
radium
intracavitary r.
radium-226 (^{226}Ra)
radius
thrombocytopenia and absent r. (TAR)
radon
radon-222 (^{222}Rn)
rales
Ramipril
Ramses
Randall stone forceps
Randall suction curette
ranitidine
rape
r. evidence
statutory r.
rape-trauma syndrome
rapid
r. bone loss
r. eye movement (REM)
r. plasma reagin (RPR)
r. slide test
rate
baseline fetal heart r.
birth r.
erythrocyte sedimentation r.
fertility r.
fetal death r.
fetal heart r. (FHR)
five-year survival r.
flow r.
glomerular filtration r. (GFR)

rate *(continued)*
heart r.
infant mortality r.
maternal death r.
maternal mortality r.
metabolic clearance r. (MCR)
mortality r.
neonatal mortality r.
ovulation r.
perinatal mortality r.
prevalence r.
sedimentation r.
sinusoidal fetal heart r.
survival r.
ventricular response r.

ratio
A/G r.
albumin/globulin ratio
amylase-creatinine clearance r.
cerebral-placental r.
cough-pressure transmission r.
estrogen/progesterone r.
fetal head:abdominal circumference r.
head:body r.
head circumference/abdominal circumference r.
L/S r.
lecithin/sphingomyelin ratio
S/D r.
sex r.
waist:hip r.

rat tooth pick-ups

ray
beta r.
gamma r.

Razoxane

Raz procedure

R band

RCGP
Royal College of General Practitioners

RDS
respiratory distress syndrome

reaction
acrosome r.
anorectic r.
Arias-Stella r.
Arthus r.
cortical r.
decidual r.
graft-versus-host r.
harlequin r.
Jarisch-Herxheimer r.
polymerase chain r. (PCR)
Porter-Silber r.
Shwartzman r.
zona r.

reactivity
fetal heart rate r.
vascular r.

reagin
rapid plasma r. (RPR)

real-time
r.-t. B-scanner
r.-t. sonography
r.-t. ultrasound

reanastomosis
tubocornual r.

rebound phenomenon

recall phenomenon

Récamier's operation

receptor
adrenergic r.
α-adrenergic r.
β-adrenergic r.
β-r. agonist
androgen r.
r. assay
class I r.
class II r.
r. coupling
endogenous opiate r.
endometrial r.
estradiol r.
estrogen r.
hormone r.
hormone complex r.
r. internalization
opiate r.
progesterone r.
steroid hormone r.

receptor-mediated endocytosis

recessive
r. disorder
r. inheritance

rechallenge

reciprocal translocation

Recklinghausen's tumor

Reclomide

recombinant
r. DNA technology
recommendation
screening r.
recommended dietary allowance
reconstruction
reconstructive
r. mammaplasty
r. surgery
record
medical r.
pregnancy r.
recorder
multichannel r.
recovery
bacterial r.
r. score
r. time
ultrasonic egg r.
recreational drug
rectal
r. cancer
r. examination
r. node
r. postradiation ulcer
rectocele
rectolabial fistula
rectosigmoid
r. colon
rectouterine
r. cul-de-sac
r. fold
r. pouch
rectovaginal
r. examination
r. fistula
r. septum
rectovestibular fistula
rectovulvar fistula
rectum
r. irradiation tolerance
recurrence
pelvic r.
r. risk
recurrent
r. abortion
r. anaphylaxis
r. carcinoma
r. genital herpes
r. infection
r. lymphoma
r. miscarriage
r. pregnancy loss
r. premenstrual lithium serum concentration decline
r. spontaneous abortion
r. vaginitis
red
r. blood cell
r. cell antigen
r. cell enzyme deficiency
r. cell volume
r. degeneration
Redisol
reducible hernia
reductase
17-ketosteroid r. deficiency
5α-reductase
reduction
embryo r.
fetal r.
limb r.
r. mammaplasty
weight r.
redundant hymen
referred pelvic pain
reflectance pulse oximetry
reflex
Ferguson r.
letdown r.
reflux
r. esophagitis
menstrual r.
r. nephropathy
refractory anemia of pregnancy
Refsum's syndrome
regeneration
tissue r.
regimen
regional
r. analgesia
r. anesthesia
r. enteritis
registry
Herbst r.
Regitine
Reglan
Regonol
regression
r. to mean
premature luteal r.
tumor r.
regulation
down r.
gonadotropin r.

regulation *(continued)*
menstrual cycle r.
physiologic follicular r.
pituitary gonadotropin r.
plasma volume r.
prolactin r.
regurgitation
aortic r.
mitral r.
Regutol
Reifenstein's syndrome
reimplantation
reinfusion
autologous bone marrow r.
Reinke's crystalloids
rejection
fetal r.
relapse
relative
r. osteopenia
r. risk
r. sterility
relaxant
muscle r.
relaxation
pelvic r.
uterine r.
relaxin
release
GnRH-facilitated FSH r.
GnRH-facilitated LH r.
gonadotropin r.
gonadotropin pulsatile r.
growth hormone r.
neurotransmitter r.
pituitary hormone r.
pulsatile r.
relief
pain r.
REM
rapid eye movement
remission
complete r.
induced r.
spontaneous r.
removal
hysteroscopic r.
renal
r. agenesis
r. artery
r. biopsy
r. calculi
r. cell carcinoma
r. cortical necrosis
r. disease
r. dysgenesis
r. failure
r. function
r. function test
r. insufficiency
r. lithiasis
r. manifestation
r. perfusion
r. plasma flow
r. stone
r. transplantation
r. tubular function
r. tubular necrosis
r. vascular thrombosis
Renese
reniform pelvis
renin
r. substrate
renin-angiotensin-aldosterone system
renin-angiotensin system
Renografin
Renoquid
repair
sphincter r.
surgical r.
vaginal r.
vaginal wall r.
vesicovaginal r.
repeat
r. cesarean
r. curettage
repeated abortion
repetitive pregnancy loss
replacement
cephalic r.
estrogen r.
fluid r.
heart valve r.
replenishment
replication fork
report
case r.
Walton r.
reproduction
assisted r.
reproductive
r. cycle
r. disorder
r. endocrinology
r. failure
r. function

r. genetics
r. history
r. mortality
r. performance
r. system
r. technology
r. tract
r. wastage
requirement
iron r.
mineral r.
nutrient r.
sodium r.
vitamin r.
rescue
abdominal r.
resectability
resection
en bloc r.
endometrial r.
laparoscopic multiple-punch r.
low rectal r.
multiple-punch r.
ovarian wedge r.
pulmonary r.
segmental r.
surgical r.
transcervical r.
transsphenoidal microsurgical r.
wedge r.
Resercen
reserpine
residual
r. ductal tissue
r. ovary syndrome
r. urine
r. urine volume
r. volume
residue
methanol extraction r. (MER)
resistance
airway r.
androgen r.
r. to antibody
bromocriptine r.
differential vascular r.
r. index
insulin r.
systemic vascular r.
total pulmonary r.
vascular r.
resistant
r. ovary
resolution
axial r.
lateral r.
resonance
nuclear magnetic r. (NMR)
resorption
bone r.
fetal r.
respiration
respiratory
r. acidosis
r. alkalosis
r. complication
r. depression
r. distress
r. distress syndrome (RDS)
r. infection
r. paralysis
r. system
r. tract
response
abnormal r.
amnestic r.
anamnestic r.
antibody r.
baroreflex r.
cortisol r.
immune r.
lactation letdown r.
maternal immune r.
maternal vascular r.
pressor r.
Rh immune r.
target organ r.
rest
bed r.
Marchand's r.
mesonephric r.
Walthard's cell r.
wolffian r.
restitution
restless legs syndrome
Restoril
restriction
r. endonuclease
r. fragment length polymorphism (RFLP)
r. site
sodium r.

resumption
menstrual cycle r.
resuscitation
cardiopulmonary r.
intrauterine r.
neonatal r.
newborn r.
Resyl
retained
r. menstruation
r. placenta
retardation
fetal growth r.
growth r.
intrauterine growth r. (IUGR)
mental r.
retarded fetal growth
rete cyst of ovary
retention
fetal r.
r. of placental tissue
reticulare
magma r.
reticulocyte count
reticulocytosis
Retin-A
retina
retinal
r. change
r. detachment
retinitis
gravidic r.
retinoblastoma
retinoic acid
retinoid
retinol
retinopathy
diabetic r.
eclamptic r.
gravidic r.
r. of prematurity
toxemic r. of pregnancy
retraction
nipple r.
r. ring
retractor
Army-Navy r.
Balfour r.
bladder r.
Deaver r.
DeLee universal r.
Gelpi perineal r.
Goulet r.
Harrington r.
Heaney-Hyst r.
Jackson right angle r.
Kelly r.
Magrina-Bookwalter vaginal r.
malleable r.
Murless head r.
r. neuropathy
O'Sullivan-O'Connor r.
Richardson r.
Roberts thumb r.
self-retaining r.
thumb r.'s
retraining
bladder r.
retrieval
oocyte r.
retrocession
retrodeviation
retrodisplacement
retroflexion, retroflection
uterine r.
retrograde
r. menstrual flow
r. menstruation
retrolental fibroplasia
retromammary mastitis
retroperitoneal
r. drain
r. endometriosis
r. infection
r. lymphadenectomy
r. node
r. soft tissue
retroperitoneum
retroplacental clot
retroposed
retroposition
retropubic
r. colpourethrocystopexy
r. space
r. urethropexy
retroversioflexion
retroversion
uterine r.
retroverted
retrovirus
Retzius' space
reversal
hyperandrogenism r.

reverse
r. transcriptase
r. triiodothyronine
Reye's syndrome
Reynolds number
RFA
right frontoanterior position
RFLP
restriction fragment length polymorphism
RFP
right frontoposterior position
RFT
right frontotransverse position
Rh
rhesus
Rh antigen
Rh blood group
Rh blood group system
Rh disease
Rh factor
Rh hemolytic disease
Rh immune response
Rh immunization
Rh isoimmunization
Rh sensitization
rhabdomyoblast
rhabdomyosarcoma
embryonal r.
Rh_0(D)
Rh_0(D) imaging
RH_0 (D) immune globulin
rhesus (Rh)
rheumatic
r. disease
r. fever
r. heart disease
rheumatoid
r. arthritis
r. vasculitis
rheumatologic disorder
Rhinall
Rhindecon
Rh-negative factor
Rh-positive
Rh-p. infant
Rh-p. red cell stroma
rhythm
circadian r.
r. method
RIA
radiommunoassay
ribavirin
riboflavin
ribonucleic
ribonucleic acid (RNA)
ribosome
Richardson retractor
Richter and Albrich procedure
ricin
rickets
vitamin D-resistant r.
ridge
cervicovaginal r.
genital r.
gonadal r.
transverse r.
Rifadin
rifampicin
rifampin
rifamycin, rifomycin
right
r. acromiodorsoposterior position
r. angle scissors
r. to be well-born
r. birthing position
r. frontoanterior position (RFA)
r. frontoposterior position (RFP)
r. frontotransverse position (RFT)
r. mentoanterior position (RMA)
r. mentoposterior position (RMP)
r. mentotransverse position (RMT)
r. occipitoanterior position (ROA)
r. occipitoposterior position (ROP)
r. occipitotransverse position (ROT)
r. ovarian vein syndrome
r. sacroanterior position (RSA)
r. sacroposterior position (RSP)
r. sacrotransverse position (RST)
right-to-left shunt
rigidity
anatomic r.
pathologic r.

Rimactane
ring
amnion r.
Bandl's r.
constriction r.
contraceptive r.
Falope r.
gestational r.
Graefenberg r.
Imlach's r.
pathologic retraction r.
r. pessary
physiologic retraction r.
progestin-impregnated vaginal r.
retraction r.
T-shaped constriction r.
tubal r.
Ringer's
lactated R.
R. solution
Rinse
Nix Cream R.
ripening
cervical r.
risk
r. factor
fetal r.
r. management
maternal r.
recurrence r.
relative r.
teratogenic r.
Ritalin
Ritgen's maneuver
ritodrine
Ritter's disease
Rivotril
RMA
right mentoanterior position
RMP
right mentoposterior position
RMT
right mentotransverse position
^{222}Rn
radon-222
RNA
ribonucleic acid
messenger R. (mRNA)
transfer R. (tRNA)
ROA
right occipitoanterior position
robertsonian
r. fusion
r. translocation
Robert's pelvis
Roberts thumb retractor
Robicillin VK
Robimycin
Robin anomalad
Robinul
Robitet
Robitussin
Rocaltrol
Rocephin
Roch-Ochs forceps
Roch-Péan forceps
rod
Gram-positive r.
Roe
roentgen (R)
roentgenography
Roe v. Wade
Roferon-A
Rohr's stria
Rokitansky
R. prominence
R. syndrome
R. tubercle
Rokitansky-Küster-Hauser syndrome
roll-over test
Rolserp
Rondomycin
rooming-in
ROP
right occipitoposterior position
Rosenmüller
organ of R.
ROT
right occipitotransverse position
rotation
r. and descent
external r.
forceps r.
internal r.
manual r.
rotational delivery
round
r. ligament
r. pelvis
round-headed acrosomeless spermatozoa
Royal College of General Practitioners (RCGP)

RPR
rapid plasma reagin
RSA
right sacroanterior position
RSP
right sacroposterior position
RST
right sacrotransverse position
RU 486
rubella
congenital r.
periconceptional r.
r. vaccination
r. vaccine
r. virus
rubeola
Rubin's maneuver
Rubin test
rudimentary uterine horn
ruga, pl. **rugae**
rule
four-hour r.
Haase's r.
His' r.
informed consent disclosure r.'s
Nägele's r.
Ogino-Knaus r.
r. of outlet
rule of 60s
rumination
Rum-K
runner's high
runt
r. disease
runting
rupture
amnion r.
corpus luteum cyst r.
hepatic r.
marginal sinus r.
membrane r.
prelabor membrane r.
premature r.
premature amnion r.
premature membrane r.
prolonged r.
splenic r.
total perineal r.
tubal r.
uterine r.
ruptured
r. cerebral aneurysm
r. episiotomy
r. membrane
r. uterus
Russian tissue forceps
Rutledge classification of extended hysterectomy
Rynacrom

Sabin vaccine
sac
amniotic s.
pseudogestational s.
small gestational s.
yolk s.
saccular
s. aneurysm
s. period
sacculation
sacral node
sacroanterior position
sacrococcygeal teratoma
sacroiliac joint
sacropexy
abdominal s.
sacroposterior position
sacrospinous ligament suspension
sacrotransverse position
sacrum
SAD
source axis distance
saddle
s. block
Saenger's operation
safe period
sagittal suture
sagrada
cascara s.
sal ammoniac
Salazopyrin
salbutamol
salicylate
choline s.
magnesium s.
sodium s.
salicylsalicylic acid
saline
s. cathartic
hypertonic s.
s. implant
normal s.
salivary gland
Salk vaccine
Salmonella typhi
salpingectomy
salpingemphraxis
salpingioma
salpingitic
salpingitis
chronic interstitial s.
foreign body s.
gonorrheal s.
granulomatous s.
s. isthmica nodosa (SIN)
leperous s.
nongranulomatous s.
pyogenic s.
tuberculous s.
salpingocele
salpingocyesis
salpingography
salpingolysis
salpingo-oophorectomy
abdominal s.-o.
bilateral s.-o. (BSO)
unilateral s.-o.
salpingo-oophoritis
salpingo-oophorocele
salpingo-ovariectomy
salpingoperitonitis
salpingopexy
salpingoplasty
salpingorrhagia
salpingorrhaphy
salpingoscopy
salpingostomatomy
salpingostomy
salpingotomy
abdominal s.
salsalate
salt
gold s.
s. wasting
Saluron
salvage therapy
sample
blood s.
sampling
blood s.
capillary blood s.
chorion s.
chorionic villus s. (CVS)
endometrial s.
fetal blood s.
fetal scalp blood s.
fetal skin s.
percutaneous blood s.

sampling *(continued)*
percutaneous umbilical blood s. (PUBS)
scalp blood s.
trophoblast s.
umbilical blood s.
Sandhoff's disease
Sandimmune
Sandostatin
sandwich assay
Sanfilippo's syndrome
Sanger incision
Sanorex
Sansert
SAP-35
saphenous nerve
sarcoidosis
sarcoma
botryoid s.
cervical s.
endometrial s.
endometrial stromal s. (ESS)
Ewing's s.
heterologous uterine s.
homologous uterine s.
Kaposi's s.
mesodermal s.
mixed mesodermal s. (MMS)
mixed müllerian s.
mixed ovarian mesodermal s.
obesity in endometrial s.
retroperitoneal soft tissue s.
uterine s.
uterine müllerian s.
vulvar s.
sarcomatous myoma degeneration
sarcomere
Sarcoptes scabiei
SART
Society for Assisted Reproductive Technology
S.A.S.-500
saturation
s. analysis
oxygen s.
Savage syndrome
saw
Gigli's s.
scabies
scalp
s. blood sampling
scan
abdominopelvic s.
iodine 125-labeled fibrinogen s.
longitudinal s.
radiofibrinogen uptake s.
time position s.
transverse s.
ventilation/perfusion s.
scanning
iodomethyl-norcholesterol s.
isotope s.
Scanzoni's
S. maneuver
S. second os
Scanzoni-Smellie maneuver
scar
lower-segment s.
perineal s.
s. prediction
radial s.
s. tissue
scarification
scarlet fever
scarred womb
scattered echo
S-C disease
sickle cell-hemoglobin C disease
Schauta vaginal operation
Schiller's
S. solution
S. test
Schilling test
schistosomiasis
schizocyte
schizocytosis
Schlusskoagulum
Schroeder
S. forceps
S. tenaculum forceps
S. vulsella forceps
Schroeder's operation
Schubert uterine biopsy forceps
Schuchardt's operation
Schultze's
S. mechanism
S. phantom
S. placenta
schwannoma
sciatic nerve
scintigraphy
ventilation s.
scirrhous carcinoma

scissors
Adson ganglion s.
bandage s.
Braun episiotomy s.
Jorgenson s.
Lister s.
Mayo s.
Mayo curved s.
Mayo straight s.
Metzenbaum s.
Metzenbaum long s.
right angle s.
Smellie's s.
straight s.
sclerocystic
s. disease of the ovary
s. ovary
scleroderma
sclero-oophoritis
sclerosing
s. adenitis
s. adenosis
s. agent
s. lesion
sclerosis, pl. **scleroses**
menstrual s.
multiple s.
ovulational s.
physiologic s.
progressive systemic s.
scoliosis
scopolamine
s. methylbromide
score
Apgar s.
Dubowitz s.
pelvic s.
recovery s.
screening
antenatal s.
antibody s.
cervical carcinoma s.
colposcopic s.
cytologic s.
genetic s.
s. laboratory tests
mammographic s.
maternal s.
prenatal s.
s. recommendation
ultrasound s.
uterine s.
S-D disease
sickle cell-hemoglobin D disease
S/D ratio
systolic/diastolic ratio
sebaceous cyst
seborrheic
s. dermatitis
s. keratosis
sebum
s. preputiale
secobarbital
Seconal
second
s. degree prolapse
s. messenger
s. parallel pelvic plane
s. pregnancy
s. stage
s. stage of labor
s. trimester
s. twin
secondary
s. abdominal pregnancy
s. amenorrhea
s. atelectasis
s. dysmenorrhea
s. infertility
s. sex characteristic
s. uterine inertia
second-look
s.-l. laparoscopy
s.-l. laparotomy
s.-l. operation
secretion
abnormal cortisol s.
adrenal androgen s.
androgen s.
follicle-stimulating hormone s.
follicular phase gonadotropin s.
gonadotropin s.
impaired s.
luteinizing hormone s.
melatonin s.
persistent estrogen s.
pituitary gonadotropin s.
placental s.
progesterone s.
prolactin s.
s. rate
steroid s.

secretion *(continued)*
syndrome of inappropriate antidiuretic hormone s.
vaginal s.
secretory
s. carcinoma
s. disease
s. IgA
s. phase
section
cesarean s. (C-section)
extraperitoneal cesarean s.
Latzko's cesarean s.
low cervical cesarean s.
transperitoneal cesarean s.
Sectral
secundigravida
secundina, pl. **secundinae**
secundines
secundipara
Sedabamate
sedation
sedative
s. effect
Sedatuss
sediment
urinary s.
sedimentation rate
segment
uterine s.
segmental resection
seizure
s. control
s. disorder
eclamptic s.
gelastic s.
Select Committee on Aging
selection
prenatal s.
selective
s. abortion
s. inguinal node dissection
s. termination
self-breast examination
self-examination
breast s.-e. (BSE)
self-monitoring
self-priming action
self-referred diagnostic imaging
self-retaining retractor
sellar enlargement
sella turcica
Sellheim incision
Sellick's maneuver
semen
s. analysis
frozen s.
s. liquefaction
s. volume
Semicid
semination
seminiferous tubule
seminoma
semiprone position
senile vaginitis
senna
Senokot
sensitivity
assay s.
sensitization
Kell s.
Rh s.
sensitizer
hypoxic cell s.
sensorineural change
sensory organ
separation
peripheral placental s.
placental s.
uterine scar s.
sepsis, pl. **sepses**
neonatal s.
postoperative s.
puerperal s.
sepsis-pneumonia syndrome
septate
s. hymen
s. uterus
septic
s. abortion
s. pelvic thrombophlebitis
s. shock
septicemia
puerperal s.
septimetritis
Septra
septum
placental s.
rectovaginal s.
transverse vaginal s.
uterine s.'s
sequela, sequelae
neoplastic s.
sequence
DNA s.

Y chromosome-specific DNA s.
sequential
s. administration
s. oral contraceptive
Serax
Sereen
Serentil
series
gastrointestinal s.
serological test
serology
seroma
postoperative s.
Seromycin
Serophene
serotonin
serous
s. adenocarcinoma
s. cystadenoma
s. tumor
Serpalan
Serpasil
Sertoli
S.'s cell
S. cell staging
S. cell tumor
Sertoli-Leydig
S.-L. cell
S.-L. cell tumor
serum
s. albumin
s. amylase
s. antibody
s. concentration
s. estrogen
fetal s.
s. HCG level
s. hepatitis
s. iron
s. level
s. levonorgestrel
s. lithium concentration
maternal s.
s. progesterone
s. prolactin
s. testosterone
s. transaminase
severe
s. fetal hydrops
sex
s. assignment
s. chromatin
chromosomal s.
s. chromosome
s. cords
s. cord-stromal germ cell tumor
s. cord stromal neoplasm
s. cord-stromal ovarian neoplasm
s. cord-stromal tumor
s. determination
s. flush
gonadal s.
s. habits
s. hormone
phenotypic s.
s. ratio
s. steroid
sex hormone-binding globulin (SHBG)
sex-linked inheritance
sexual
s. abuse
s. activity
s. ambiguity
s. assault
s. derivation
s. differentiation
s. dysfunction
s. experience
s. function
s. hair
s. history
s. intercourse
s. molestation
s. partner
s. response curve
s. response cycle
s. transmission
sexually transmitted disease (STD)
SGO
Society of Gynecologic Oncology
shake test
Shauta-Aumreich procedure
SHBG
sex hormone-binding globulin
sheath
fibrin s.
shedding
asymptomatic viral s.
Sheehan's syndrome
sheet
amniotic s.

shield
- Dalkon s.
- nipple s.

shift
- Doppler s.
- luteoplacental s.

Shigella

shigellosis

Shirodkar
- S. cervical cerclage
- S. operation
- S. procedure

shock
- cardiogenic s.
- hemorrhagic s.
- hypovolemic s.
- peripheral vascular s.
- postoperative s.
- septic s.
- toxic s.

short-axis view

short-limb dystrophy

short luteal phase

short-term increase

shoulder
- s. dystocia
- s. pain
- s. presentation

show
- bloody s.

shunt
- left-to-right s.
- right-to-left s.
- ventriculoperitoneal s.

Shur-Seal

Shute forceps

Shwartzman reaction

sialic acid

sialorrhea

sicca syndrome

sicchasia

sickle
- s. cell anemia
- s. cell crisis
- s. cell disease
- s. cell-hemoglobin C disease (S-C disease)
- s. cell-hemoglobin D disease (S-D disease)
- s. cell-hemoglobin S disease
- s. cell-β-thalassemia disease
- s. cell trait

sickness
- morning s.

SIDS
- sudden infant death syndrome

sigmoid colon

sigmoiditis

sigmoidoscopy

sign
- Braxton-Hicks s.
- Calkins' s.
- Chadwick's s.
- Cullen's s.
- Danforth's s.
- double bubble s.
- Gauss' s.
- Goodell's s.
- Gower's s.
- groove s.
- halo s.
- halo s. of hydrops
- Hartman's s.
- Hegar's s.
- Homans' s.
- jello s.
- lemon s.
- placental s.
- Spalding's s.
- turtle s.
- vital s.

signal
- abnormal feedback s.'s

signet ring cell carcinoma

Silastic cup extractor

silent
- s. amnionitis
- s. fetal heart rate pattern
- s. pelvic inflammatory disease

silicone
- s. implant
- s. implant leakage
- s. injection
- s. plug

silk suture

silver
- s. nitrate
- s. wire suture

Silver's syndrome

simethicone

Simmonds' disease

Simon's position

simple
- s. colloid goiter

s. cyst
s. mastectomy
s. urethritis
s. vulvectomy
Simpson
S. uterine sound
Simpson's forceps
Sims
S. curette
S. position
S. uterine sound
simulation
SIN
salpingitis isthmica nodosa
sincipital presentation
sinciput
Sinequan
single
s. intrauterine death
s. kidney
single-dose methotrexate therapy
single-gene defect
single-photon absorptiometry
singleton pregnancy
single-tooth tenaculum
Singley forceps
sinovaginal bulb
Sinufed
sinus, pl. **sinus, sinuses**
s. bradycardia
s. tachycardia
urogenital s.
uterine s.
uteroplacental s.
sinusoid
sinusoidal fetal heart rate
sirenomelia
sister chromatid
site
antibody reaction s.
antigen binding s.
binding s.
bleeding s.
placental s.
placental bleeding s.
restriction s.
in situ
in situ carcinoma of vagina
sitz bath
sixth disease
size
corpus luteum s.
focal spot s.
maternal s.
small sac s.
tumor s.
uterine s.
Sjögren-Larsson syndrome
Sjögren's syndrome
SK-Amitriptyline
skeletal
s. abnormality
s. calcium deficiency
s. dysplasia
s. growth
s. maturation
Skene's
S. duct
S. gland
skin
s. atrophy
s. calcification
s. disease
s. lesion
s. pore
s. tag
s. test
s. thickening
s. trigger theory
vulvar s.
skinning vulvectomy
skip area
SK-pramine
skull fracture
SLE
systemic lupus erythematosus
sleep
twilight s.
sliding
s. hernia
s. lock
sling procedure
Slo-Phyllin
Slow K
slow-release sodium fluoride
Slow-Trasicor
small
s. bowel
s. gestational sac
s. intestine decompression
s. sac size
small-for-gestational-age infant
smallpox
s. vaccine
Smead-Jones closure

smear
cervical s.
Pap s.
wet s.
smegma
s. clitoridis
s. preputii
Smellie's scissors
Smith-Hodge pessary
Smith-Lemli-Opitz syndrome
smoke
s. inhalation
smooth
s. muscle
SMZ-TMP
trimethoprim-sulfamethoxazole
snowflake pattern
snuffles
soap
Basis s.
social
s. factor
s. history
Society
S. for Assisted Reproductive Technology (SART)
S. of Gynecologic Oncology (SGO)
S. for Gynecologic Pathology
socioeconomic status
sodium
s. balance
s. bicarbonate
s. bromide
cefoxitin s.
s. chloride
s. chloride slide
s. citrate with citric acid
cromolyn s.
s. cyclamate
s. diatrizoate
docusate s.
s. excretion
s. fluoride
heparin s.
s. iodide
s. iodide I 125
s. iodide I 131
s. nitroprusside
s. requirement
s. restriction
s. salicylate
thiopental s.
s. thiosulfate
zomepirac s.
Sodium Sulamyd
softener
stool s.
soft tissue
soft-tissue ovarian neoplasm
Solatene
Solazine
Solfoton
Solganal
solid-phase enzyme immunoassay
solitary
s. dilated duct
s. kidney
Solium
soluble antigen
solution
Bouin's s.
Burow's s.
lactated Ringer's s.
Lugol's iodine s.
Monsel's s.
Ringer's s.
Schiller's s.
somatic nervous system feedback loop
somatomedin C
somatostatin
somatotrope
somatotropinoma
somite formation
Somophyllin
sonographic finding
sonography
real-time s.
transvaginal s.
vaginal s.
sonolucent tissue
Sorbitrate
sorter
fluorescent-activated cell s. (FACS)
souffle
fetal s.
funic s., funicular s.
mammary s.
placental s.
umbilical s.
uterine s.
sound
bowel s.'s

fetal heart s.
heart s.
Simpson uterine s.
Sims uterine s.
uterine s.

sound-stimulated fetal movement
source axis distance (SAD)
source-to-skin distance (SSD)
Southern blot
Soyacal
space
intervillous s.'s
s. medicine
Retzius' s.
subchorial s.

Spalding's sign
span
fertilizable life s.

Sparine
sparing
brain s.

spasm
infantile s.
levator ani s.
urethral s.

spasmodic dysmenorrhea
spatula
Ayers s.
s. cytobrush

species
specific
s. immunotherapy
s. urethritis

specificity
assay s.

specimen
midstream urine s.

spectinomycin
Spectrobid
spectrophotometry
spectrum
electromagnetic s.

specular echo
speculum, pl. **specula**
Auvard s.
bivalve s.
duckbill s.
s. examination
Graves bivalve s.
Pedersen's s.
weighted s.

Spence
axillary tail of S.
S. axillary tail
S. and Duckett marsupialization

sperm
s. allergy
s. antibody
s. attrition
s. capacitation
s. count
s. donation
donor s.
epididymal s.
s. immobilization test
s. penetration assay

spermatocide
spermatogenesis
spermatogonia
spermatozoa
round-headed acrosomeless s.
washed s.

spermatozoan penetration
spermicide
spermidine
spermine
sperm-oocyte interaction
Spersacarpine
S phase fraction
spherocytosis
hereditary s.

sphincter
s. repair
urethral s.
s. weakness

sphingomyelin
spiculated lesion
spider
s. angioma
s. nevus
vascular s.

Spiegelberg's criteria
spigelian hernia
spina bifida
spina bifida cystica
spina bifida occulta
spinal
s. analgesia
s. anesthesia
s. angioma
s. blockade
s. bone loss
s. compression fracture
s. cord

spinal *(continued)*
- s. headache
- s. injury
- s. quantitative computerized tomography

spindle cell sarcoma of vagina

spine

Spinelli operation

spinnbarkeit

spiral
- s. artery
- s. electrode

spiramycin

spirochete

spironolactone

splanchnic pelvic pain

spleen

splenectomy

splenic
- s. pregnancy
- s. rupture
- s. sequestration syndrome
- s. tissue
- s. torsion

splenosis

split-thickness graft

splitting
- muscle s.

spondylitis
- ankylosing s.

sponge
- absorbable gelatin s.
- contraceptive s.
- s. forceps
- s. holding forceps
- intravaginal s.
- s. sticks
- vaginal s.

spontaneous
- s. abortion
- s. amputation
- s. cephalic delivery
- s. evolution
- s. gangrene of newborn
- s. menstrual cycle
- s. ovulation
- s. preterm delivery
- s. remission
- s. rupture of membrane
- s. version

spot
- blood s.'s
- café au lait s.
- s. compression
- s. compression view
- s. magnification
- strawberry s.

spread
- Halstedian concept of tumor s.
- vessel s.

sprout
- syncytial s.

spurious pregnancy

squama

squamocolumnar junction

squamous
- s. cell
- s. cell carcinoma
- s. epithelium
- s. metaplasia

square
- chi-s. (χ^2)

Sα-reductase

SSD

source-to-skin distance

SS disease

stabilization

stab wound

Stadol

stage
- cortical supremacy s.
- delayed first s.
- diakinesis s.
- dictyate s.
- indifferent gonadal s.
- s.'s of labor
- leptotene s.
- pachytene s.
- placental s.
- zygotene s.

stages of labor

Staging
- American Joint Committee for Cancer S. (AJCC)

staging
- clinical s.
- surgical s.
- Tanner s.

stagnation mastitis

stain
- Betke s.
- Feulgen s.
- Giemsa s.
- Gram's s.
- iodine s.

Kleihauer-Betke s.
meconium s.
Wright's s.
staining
blood pigment s.
meconium s.
stainless steel suture
stalk
body s.
infundibular s.
Stamey's modification of Pereyra procedure
stance
Buddha s.
standard
s. curve
s. deviation
ethical s.
protein s.
Stanley Way procedure
Staphcillin
Staphylococcus
S. aureus
S. saprophyticus
staphylococcus
staple
absorbable s.
star effect
starvation
accelerated s.
s. ketosis
state
accompanying mood s.
menstrual s.
mood s.
state-of-the-art radiation
static B-scanner
station
0 s.
fetal s.
statistical term
Statobex
stature
maternal s.
status
acid-base s.
s. epilepticus
Karnofsky performance s.
s. lymphaticus
socioeconomic s.
s. thymicolymphaticus
s. thymicus
statutory rape
STD
sexually transmitted disease
Stein-Leventhal
S.-L. syndrome
Stelazine
stellate mass
stem cell assay
Stemetil
stenosis
aortic s.
aqueductal s.
cervical s.
idiopathic hypertrophic subaortic s.
mitral s.
pulmonary s.
pyloric s.
renal artery s.
subaortic s.
stent
double J s.
urinary s.
stereocolpogram
stereocolposcope
stereoscopic pelvimetry
stereotaxis
sterile
s. pyuria syndrome
sterility
absolute s.
adolescent s.
one-child s.
relative s.
sterilization
intermittent s.
involuntary s.
tubal s.
voluntary s.
sterilize
steroid
adrenal s.
adrenocortical s.
s. biosynthesis
s. cell
s. concentration
s. contraceptive
endogenous s.
s. hormone
17-ketogenic s.
long-acting contraceptive s.
s. metabolism
s. metabolite
s. nucleus

steroid *(continued)*
ovarian s.
placental s.
s. receptor
s. secretion
sex s.
s. sulfatase
s. therapy
steroidogenesis
adrenocortical s.
fetal-placental s.
follicle s.
ovarian s.
testicular s.
Stewart-Treves syndrome
S-thalassemia disease
stick
sponge s.'s
stigma
stilbestrol
stillbirth
s. rate
stillborn infant
Still's disease
stimulant
stimulation
cervical carcinoma s.
endometrial s.
exogenous gonadotropin s.
follicle maturation s.
ovulation s.
oxytocic s.
prolactin s.
s. test
vibroacoustic s.
stimulator
adrenergic s.
alpha-adrenergic s.
hematopoietic system s.
long-acting thyroid s. (LATS)
luteinization s.
stitch
McCall s.
Stockholm technique for radium therapy
stocking
antiembolism s.
elastic s.
leg-compression s.'s
stomach cancer
stomatomy
stomatotomy
stone
kidney s.
renal s.
stool
s. examination
s. softener
storm
thyroid s.
Stoxil
straight
s. catheter test
s. scissors
strait
inferior s.
superior s.
strangulated hernia
strangulation
small bowel s.
Strassman
S. metroplasty
S. phenomenon
S. technique
transverse fundal incision of S.
stratified squamous epithelium
stratum, gen. **strati**, pl. **strata**
s. basale
s. compactum
s. functionale
strawberry appearance
strawberry spot
streak
gonadal s.
primitive s.
Strema
Streptase
streptococcal
s. infection
s. vaginitis
Streptococcus
S. milleri
S. pneumoniae
streptococcus, pl. **streptococci**
group A s.
group B s.
group D streptococcus
β-hemolytic s.
streptokinase
streptokinase-urokinase
streptomycin
stress
emotional s.
s. incontinence

life s.
maternal s.
postmenstrual s.
psychological s.
s. reaction
s. test
s. urinary incontinence
stressed fetus
stria, gen. and pl. **striae**
abdominal s.
striae atrophicae
striae cutis distensae
striae gravidarum
Langhans' s.
Rohr's s.
striated muscle
strip
fascial s.
Mersilene fascial s.
polypropylene fascial s.
Stroganoff's method
stroke
stroma
cervical s.
fibromuscular cervical s.
gonadal s.
ovarian s.
Rh-positive red cell s.
uterine endolymphatic s.
uterine endometrial s.
uterine epithelial s.
stromal
s. hyperthecosis
s. microinvasion
stromatosis
strontium bromide
struma, pl. **strumae**
s. ovarii
strumal carcinoid
Stuart index
Study
Intergroup Rhabdomyosarcoma S. (IRS)
Oxford Family Planning Association Contraceptive S.
Royal College of General Practioners' Oral Contraception S.
study
acoustic stimulation s.
barium s.
biochemical s.
blood s.
CASH s.
cytogenetic s.
fetal blood s.
histopathological s.
maternal blood s.
postmortem s.
tissue s.
urodynamic s.
Sturmdorf hemostatic suture
Sturmdorf's operation
stype
subaortic
s. node
s. stenosis
subarachnoid
s. block
s. hemorrhage
subareolar duct papillomatosis
subchorial
s. lake
s. space
subchorionic hemorrhage
subclavian thrombosis
subclinical hypothyroidism
subcutaneous mastectomy
subdermal implant
subfertility
subfragment-1
subinvolution
Sublimaze
submammary mastitis
submucosal
s. myoma
s. plexus
submucous
s. leiomyoma
s. myoma
subnuclear
s. vacuole
s. vacuolization
suboccipitobregmatic diameter
suboptimal surgery
subpectoral implant
subseptate uterus
subsequent fertility
subserous, subserosal
s. fascia
s. myoma
substance
müllerian-inhibiting s.
substance P

substrate
renin s.
subtotal hysterectomy
subunit
α-subunit
β-subunit
succenturiate placenta
successful pregnancy
succinylcholine
succinylsulfathiazole
suckle
suckling
suction
airway s.
s. catheter
s. curettage
s. drainage
nasopharyngeal s.
Vabra s.
suctioning
DeLee s.
Sudafed
sudden infant death syndrome (SIDS)
Sudrin
sufentanil citrate
sugar
blood s.
suicide
suit
malpractice s.
Sulf-10
sulfa
sulfacarbamide
sulfacetamide
sulfachlorpyridazine
sulfacytine
sulfadiazine
sulfadimethoxine
sulfadimidine
sulfadoxine
sulfaethidole
sulfafurazole, sulphafurazole
sulfaguanidine
sulfalene
sulfamerazine
sulfameter
sulfamethazine
sulfamethizole
sulfamethoxazole
sulfamethoxydiazine
sulfamethoxypyridazine
Sulfamylon
sulfanilamide
sulfaphenazole, sulphaphenazole
sulfa preparation
sulfapyridine
sulfasalazine
sulfatase
steroid s.
sulfate
dehydroepiandrosterone s. (DHEAS)
dehydroisoandrosterone s.
ephedrine s.
ferric s.
ferrous s.
magnesium s.
metaproterenol s.
orciprenaline s.
piperazine estrone s.
terbutaline s.
sulfathiazole
sulfathiourea
sulfisomidine
sulfisoxazole
sulfonamide
sulfonate
2-mercaptoethane s. (MESNA)
sulfonylurea
sulfotransferase
estrogen s.
sulfur granule
sulindac
sulphafurazole
sulpiride
summary
discharge s.
Sumycin
superfecundation
superfetation
superficial
s. spreading melanoma
s. thrombophlebitis
superimposed
s. eclampsia
s. preeclampsia
superimpregnation
superinvolution
superior
s. mesenteric artery
s. mesenteric plexus
s. vena cava
s. vena caval syndrome
superlactation

supernumerary
s. mamma
s. ovary
s. placenta
superovulation
s. induction
superumbilical incision
supervoltage
s. radiation
supine
s. hypotensive syndrome
s. position
s. pressor test
supplement
calcium s.
vitamin s.
supplementary menstruation
supplementation
calcium s.
supply
iodine s.
support
s. group
psychosocial s.
suppository
prostaglandin s.
vaginal s.
suppressed menstruation
suppression
endogenous gonadotropin activity s.
estradiol s.
gonadal steroid s.
immunologic s.
pituitary gonadotropin s.
prolactin s.
testosterone s.
suppressor
s. cell
s. T cell
suppuration
suppurative
s. mastitis
s. phlebitis
supracervical hysterectomy
suprapubic
s. cystotomy
s. pain
s. urethrovesical suspension operation
supraumbilical incision
supraventricular
s. tachycardia
s. tachydysrhythmia (SVT)
surface
s. antigen
s. epithelium
s. immunoglobulin
s. irradiation
surfactant
surge
estrogen s.
midcycle s.
preovulatory LH s.
surgery
bariatric s.
bypass s.
conservative s.
cytoreductive s.
fetal s.
gastric reduction s.
hysteroscopic s.
inadequate s.
intra-abdominal s.
laser s.
maternal s.
palliative s.
pelvic s.
pelvic-floor s.
radical s.
suboptimal s.
tubal reconstruction s.
vaginal s.
surgical
s. infection
s. management
s. reconstruction
s. repair
s. resection
s. staging
s. weight loss
surgically induced abortion
Surmontil
surrogate
surveillance
fetal s.
immunologic s.
maternal s.
nutritional s.
s. technique
ultrasound s.
10-year s.
Survey
Third National Cancer S.

survival
actuarial s.
allograft s.
life table s.
long-term s.
s. rate
susceptibility
genetic s.
suspension
bladder neck s.
Coffey s.
minimal-incision pubovaginal s.
sacrospinous ligament s.
uterine s.
suspensory
s. ligament of the ovary
s. sling operation
Sus-Phrine
Sustaire
sutural calcification
suture
absorbable s.
catgut s.
continuous running monofilament s.
Dexon s.
gut s.
s. material
Mersilene s.
polygalactide s.
polyglycol s.
polyglyconate s.
purse-string s.
sagittal s.
silk s.
silver wire s.
stainless steel s.
Sturmdorf hemostatic s.
Vicryl s.
suturing
peritoneal s.
SVT
supraventricular tachydysrhythmia
swallowing
fetal s.
Swan-Ganz catheter
swelling
labioscrotal s.
Swiss cheese endometrium
Swyer's syndrome
Symmetrel
symmetric communicating uterus
sympathectomy, sympathetectomy
presacral s.
sympathetic nervous system
sympathomimetic
symphysiotome, symphyseotome
symphysiotomy, symphyseotomy
symphysis pubis
symptom
premenstrual s.'s
symptomatic infection
symptoms
sympto-thermal method
Synalar
Synalgos-DC
synapsis
Synarel
Synasal
synchondrotomy
synclitic
synclitism
syncytial
s. bud
s. knot
s. sprout
syncytiotrophoblast
malignant s.
syncytium
syndrome
Aase s.
acid aspiration s.
acquired immunodeficiency s. (AIDS)
acute urethral s.
adrenal virilizing s.
adrenogenital s.
adult respiratory distress s. (ARDS)
Ahumada-Del Castillo s.
air leak s.
Allen-Masters s.
amenorrhea-galactorrhea s.
amniotic fluid s.
androgen-insensitive s.
androgen insensitivity s.
Argonz-Del Castillo s.
Asherman's s.
battered fetus s.
battered wife s.
Beckwith-Wiedemann s.
Bloom's s.
brain-death s.

burning vulvar s.
carpal tunnel s.
cat-cry s.
caudal regression s.
Chiari-Frommel s.
climacteric s.
clomiphene-resistant polycystic ovary s.
congenital rubella s.
contiguous gene s.
corpus luteum deficiency s.
cri-du-chat s.
Curtis s.
Cushing's s.
Dandy-Walker s.
dead fetus s.
DiGeorge s.
Down's s.
dwarf s.
dysmaturity s.
dysuria-sterile pyuria s.
Edwards' s.
Ehlers-Danlos s.
Eisenmenger s.
Ellis-van Creveld s.
empty scrotum s.
empty sella s.
extended rubella s.
Fanconi's s.
Felty's s.
feminization s.
fetal alcohol s.
fetal aspiration s.
fetal hydantoin s.
fetal phenytoin s.
fetal trimethadione s.
fetal warfarin s.
feto-fetal transfusion s.
fibrinogen-fibrin conversion s.
Fitz-Hugh and Curtis s.
fragile X s.
gonadotrophin-resistant ovary s.
gray s., gray baby s.
Halban's s.
HELLP s.
hemolytic uremic s.
Holt-Oram s.
Hunter's s.
Hurler's s.
21-hydroxylase deficiency s.
hyperandrogenism, insulin resistance, acanthosis nigricans s.
hyperviscosity s.
immunodeficiency s.
s. of inappropriate antidiuretic hormone secretion
insensitive ovary s.
Kallmann's s.
Kartagener's s.
Klinefelter's s.
Laurence-Moon-Bardet-Biedl s.
Lesch-Nyhan s.
Li-Fraumeni cancer s.
Lub's s.
lupus obstetric s.
luteinized unruptured follicle s.
Marañón's s.
Marfan's s.
Maroteaux-Lamy s.
maternal hydrops s.
Mayer-Rokitansky-Küster-Hauser s.
McCune-Albright s.
McKusick-Kaufman s.
Meadows' s.
meconium aspiration s.
meconium blockage s.
Meigs' s.
Mendelson's s.
Menkes' s.
menopausal s.
Miller-Dieker s.
neonatal respiratory distress s.
nephrotic s.
Noonan's s.
ovarian hyperstimulation s.
ovarian remnant s.
overdistention s.
Patau's s.
pelvic congestion s.
Peutz-Jeghers s.
Pierre Robin s.
placental dysfunction s.
polycystic ovary s. (PCOS)
polyglandular s.
postmaturity s.
postmenopausal s.

syndrome *(continued)*
postpartum hemolytic uremic s.
postpartum pituitary necrosis s.
postrubella s.
post-tubal ligation s.
Potter's s.
Prader-Willi s.
premenstrual s. (PMS)
premenstrual salivary s.
premenstrual tension s.
primary empty sella s.
pulmonary dysmaturity s.
rape-trauma s.
Refsum's s.
Reifenstein's s.
residual ovary s.
resistant ovary s.
respiratory distress s. (RDS)
respiratory distress s. of the newborn
restless legs s.
Reye's s.
right ovarian vein s.
Rokitansky-Küster-Hauser s.
Sanfilippo's s.
Savage s.
sepsis-pneumonia s.
Sheehan's s.
sicca s.
Silver's s.
Sjögren-Larsson s.
Sjögren's s.
Smith-Lemli-Opitz s.
splenic sequestration s.
Stein-Leventhal s.
sterile pyuria s.
Stewart-Treves s.
sudden infant death s. (SIDS)
superior vena caval s.
supine hypotensive s.
Swyer's s.
terminal Xp deletion s.
testicular feminization s.
thoracic compression s.
thyrohypophysial s.
Tietze's s.
TORCH s.
toxic shock s. (TSS)
trichorhinophalangeal s.
triple X s.
Turner's s.
universal joint s.
urethral s.
uterine hernia s.
VACTERL s.
vanishing testes s.
vanishing twin s.
von Willebrand's s.
West's s.
Wilson-Mikity s.
Wolff-Parkinson-White s.
Wolfram's s.
45,X s.
XX male s.
47,XXX s.
47,XXY s.
XYY s.
YY s.

synechia, pl. **synechiae**
intrauterine s.

syngeneic tissue

syngraft

Synkayvite

Synodroy

Synophylate

synthase
prostaglandin s.

synthesis
decidual prolactin s.
estrogen s.
ovarian estrogen s.
progesterone s.

synthetic suture material

Synthroid

Syntocinon

syphilis
congenital s.
s. hereditaria, hereditary s.
s. hereditaria tarda

syringe
Asepto s.

syringoma

system
ABO blood group s.
autonomic nervous s.
Bethesda s.
bicarbonate-carbonic acid s.
bursa-dependent s.
cardiovascular s.
CDE blood group s.
central nervous s. (CNS)
digestive s.
endocrine s.

Ferriman and Gallwey hirsutism scoring s.
fibrinolytic and clotting s.
image recording s.
immune s.
Kagan staging s.
male reproductive s.
musculoskeletal s.
nervous s.
neuroendocrine s.
parasympathetic nervous s.
prognostic scoring s.
prorenin-renin-angiotensin s.
renin-angiotensin s.
renin-angiotensin-aldosterone s.
reproductive s.
respiratory s.
Rh blood group s.
selective no-fault s.
sympathetic nervous s.
urinary s.

systemic
s. illness
s. lupus erythematosus (SLE)
s. vascular resistance

systemic-active nonspecific immunotherapy

systolic/diastolic ratio (S/D ratio)

systolic murmur

Syva test

T

T
T band
T cell
T lymphocyte
T_3
triiodothyronine
T_4
thyroxine
^{182}Ta
tantalum-182
TAA
tumor-associated antigen
table
Bayley-Pinneau t.
height t.
tablets
hormonal pregnancy test t.
TACE
tachyarrhythmia
tachycardia
sinus t.
supraventricular t.
ventricular t.
tachydysrhythmia
supraventricular t. (SVT)
tachypnea
transient t.
tactile sensory monitoring
TAF
tumor angiogenesis factor
tag
skin t.
Tagamet
TAH
total abdominal hysterectomy
tail
axillary t.
Spence axillary t.
taking
history t.
talc
talipes
t. equinovarus
Talwin
Tambocor
tamoxifen citrate
tampon
vaginal t.
Tanner
T. stage
T. staging
tantalum
tantalum-182 (^{182}Ta)
tanycyte
Tao
Tapar
Tapazole
tapiroid
TAR
thrombocytopenia and absent radius
Taractan
Tarasan
target
t. cell
molybdenum t.
t. organ response
tungsten t.
Tarnier's
T. axis-traction forceps
tartrate
ergotamine t.
metoprolol t.
taste bud
taurine
tautomenial
Tavist
taxis
bipolar t.
taxol
Tay-Sachs disease
TBG
thyroid-binding globulin
TBP
thyroxine-binding protein
TDLU
terminal duct lobular unit
tdy gene
TE
thromboembolic disease
Tebrazid
technetium
technique
balloon catheter t.
clip t.
contraceptive t.
double-freeze t.
Eklund t.

technique *(continued)*
evoked potential t.
ferning t.
hybridoma t.
immune monitoring t.
immune separation t.
insemination swim-up t.
Jones and Jones wedge t.
Kehr t.
Krönig t.
Lapides t.
marsupialization t.
modified Pomeroy t.
molecular genetic t.
Southern blot t.
Strassman t.
surveillance t.
Tompkins median bivalving t.
tubal ligation band t.
Technology
Society for Assisted Reproductive T. (SART)
technology
recombinant DNA t.
reproductive t.
Teflon periurethral injection
Tegison
Tegopen
Tegretol
telangiectasia
ataxia t.
Teldrin
teleologic theory
teletherapy
TeLinde operation
telogen
t. effluvium
t. phase
telophase
Temaril
temazepam
temperature
basal body t.
temporary diverting colostomy
Tempra
tenaculum
Braun-Schroeder single-tooth t.
double-tooth t.
Jacobs t.
Schroeder t.
Schroeder uterine t.
single-tooth t.
tendency
familial t.
tenderness
lower abdominal t.
pelvic t.
Tenex
teniposide
Tenol
Tenoretic
Tenormin
Tensilon
tension
carbon dioxide t.
t. cyst
oxygen t.
premenstrual t.
tent
intracervical t.
laminaria t.
Tenuate
Tepanil
teratoblastoma
teratocarcinoma
teratogen
teratogenesis
teratogenic
t. agent
t. effect
t. outcome
t. risk
teratogenicity
teratology
teratoma
benign cystic ovarian t.
immature ovarian t.
malignant t.
malignant ovarian t.
mature cystic ovarian t.
mature ovarian t.
ovarian t.
ovarian cystic t.
ovarian embryonal t.
pediatric ovarian t.
sacrococcygeal t.
teratophobia
teratospermia
Terazol
terbutaline
t. sulfate
terconazole
Terfluzine

term
- t. gestation
- t. infant
- statistical t.

Term-Guard

terminal
- t. duct lobular unit (TDLU)
- t. hair
- t. neosalpingostomy
- t. saccular period
- t. Xp deletion syndrome

termination
- selective t.

terminus
- vaginal t.

Terramycin

TEST
- tubal embryo stage transfer

test
- ACTH stimulation t.
- agglutination t.
- antiglobulin t.
- antitreponemal t.
- A.-Z. t.
- A.-Z. t.
  - Aschheim-Zondek test
- Betke-Kleihauer t.
- bladder muscle stress t.
- bladder neck elevation t.
- blood-type t.
- Bonney's t.
- bubble stability t.
- coagulation t.
- contraction stress t.
- Coombs' t.
- dehydroepiandrosterone sulfate loading t.
- dexamethasone suppression t.
- early pregnancy t.
- endocrine t.
- estrogen-progestin t.
- fern t.
- fetal acoustic stimulation t.
- fetal activity t.
- fluorescein-conjugated monoclonal antibody t.
- fluorescent treponemal antibody-absorption t.
- foam stability t.
- Franklin-Dukes t.
- Frei t.
- Friberg microsurgical agglutination t.
- Friedman t.
- Friedman rabbit t.
- gelatin agglutination t.
- glucose challenge t.
- glucose tolerance t.
- gonozyme t.
- guaiac t.
- hemagglutination treponemal t. (HATTS)
- heparin challenge t.
- Huhner t.
- human ovum fertilization t.
- Immunobead t.
- immunofluorescent antibody t.
- immunologic pregnancy t.
- insulin tolerance t.
- Kibrick t.
- Kleihauer-Betke t.
- laboratory t.
- latex fixation t.
- LH Color t.
- Liddle's t.
- liver function t.
- Lumadex-FSI t.
- Marchetti t.
- metyrapone t.
- MicroTrak t.
- nipple stimulation t.
- nitrazine t.
- nonstress t.
- one-hour glucose tolerance t.
- one-tail t.
- oxytocin challenge t. (OCT)
- phenolsulfonphthalein t.
- platelet function t.
- postcoital t.
- predictive value of t.
- predictive value of negative t.
- predictive value of positive t.
- pregnancy t.
- progesterone challenge t.
- pulmonary function t.'s
- Q-tip t.
- rapid plasma reagin t.
- rapid plasma reagin card t.
- rapid slide t.
- renal function t.

test *(continued)*
roll-over t.
Rubin t.
Schiller's t.
Schilling t.
screening laboratory t.'s
serological t.
shake t.
skin t.
sperm immobilization t.
stimulation t.
straight catheter t.
stress t.
supine pressor t.
Syva t.
thrombin clot t.
thyrotropin-releasing hormone stimulation t.
tilt t.
tissue thromboplastin-inhibition t.
toluidine blue t.
TPI t.
Treponema pallidum immobilization t.
two-tail t.
urinary concentration t.
urine t.
Venereal Disease Research Laboratory t.
Western blot t.
whiff t.
withdrawal bleeding t.
zona-free hamster egg penetration t.
Zondek-Aschheim t.

testes-determining factor

testicular
t. cancer
t. differentiation
t. feminization
t. steroidogenesis

testing
ambulatory uterine contraction t.
enzyme-linked antiglobulin t.
HIV t.
home pregnancy t.
routine preoperative t.

testis, pl. **testes**
gonadotropin-resistant t.

testolactone

testosterone
bound t.
free t.
t. index
non-sex hormone-binding globulin bound t.
plasma t.
serum t.
t. suppression
topical t.

testosterone-estrogen-binding globulin

testosterone-secreting
t.-s. adrenal adenoma

test-tube baby

TET
tubal embryo transfer

tetania
t. gravidarum
t. neonatorium

tetanism

tetanus
t. immune globulin
t. neonatorum
postpartum t.
puerperal t.
t. toxoid
t. toxoid booster
uterine t.

tetany
neonatal t.

tetrabenazine

tetracaine hydrochloride

tetracycline
t. analogue
t. pleurodesis
prophylactic t.

Tetracyn

tetrad

9-tetrahydrocannabinol (THC)

tetrahydrocortisol

tetralogy of Fallot

tetranitrate
erythrityl t.
pentaerythritol t.

tetraploid distribution

tetraploidy

TGFα
transforming growth factor alpha

TGFβ
transforming growth factor beta

thalassemia

α-thalassemia

β-thalassemia
α-thalassemia intermedia
thalassemic
thalidomide
thanatophoric
THC
    9-tetrahydrocannabinol
theca
    t. cell
    t. externa
    t. interna
    t. lutein cell
    t. lutein cyst
theca-granulosa cell cooperativity
thecal/interstitial cell
thecoma
    luteinized t.
    ovarian t.
thelarche
    premature t.
theleplasty
theloncus
thelorrhagia
Theobid
Theoclear
Theo-Dur
Theolair
Theon
theophyllinate
    choline t.
theophylline
theory
    clonal selection t.
    endorphin, dopamine, and prostaglandin t.
    ganglion trigger t.
    grandmother t.
    implantation t.
    skin trigger t.
    teleologic t.
Theostat
Theovent
therapeutic
    t. abortion
    t. insemination
    t. window
therapy
    adjuvant t.
    antibacterial t.
    anticoagulant t.
    antidepressant t.
    antiemetic t.
    antifungal drug t.
    antihelminthic t.
    antihypertensive t.
    antimicrobial t.
    antiparasitic drug t.
    antithyroid drug t.
    antiviral t.
    biofeedback t.
    blood component t.
    bromocriptine t.
    cancer t.
    electroshock t.
    embolization t.
    erythromycin t.
    estrogen t.
    estrogen-progestin replacement t.
    estrogen replacement t.
    extended field irradiation t.
    external radiation t.
    external x-ray t.
    fetal drug t.
    fluid t.
    gene t.
    glucocorticosteroid t.
    gold t.
    hormonal antineoplastic t.
    hormone t.
    hormone replacement t.
    immunosuppressive t.
    internal radiation t.
    interstitial t.
    intraperitoneal t.
    intraperitoneal radiation t.
    iodide t.
    laser t.
    menopausal estrogen replacement t.
    monoclonal antibody t.
    neutron t.
    oral hormone replacement t.
    photodynamic t.
    polyvalent immunoglobulin t.
    postmenopausal estrogen t.
    postmenopausal estrogen replacement t.
    progestational t.
    progestogen support t.
    radiation t.
    salvage t.
    single-dose methotrexate t.
    steroid t.
    thrombolytic t.

therapy *(continued)*
L-thyroxine t.
tocolytic t.
transdermal hormone replacement t.
vaginal estrogen t.
vasopressin t.
x-ray t.
thermal injury
thermography
thermoregulation
thiabendazole
thiamine
thiazide
t. diuretic
thickening
skin t.
thickness
endometrial t.
placental t.
thin-layer chromatography
thioguanine
thiomalate
gold sodium t.
thiopental sodium
thiopropazate
thioridazine hydrochloride
thiosulfate
sodium t.
Thiosulfil
thiotepa
thiothixene
thiphenamil hydrochloride
third
t. degree prolapse
t. parallel pelvic plane
t. stage of labor
t. trimester
Third National Cancer Survey
Thomas curette
Thomas-Gaylor biopsy forceps
thoracic
t. clamp
t. compression syndrome
thoracolumbar sympathetic nerve
thorax
Thorazine
threatened
t. abortion
t. miscarriage
threshold trait
thrive
failure to t.
thrombectomy
thrombi
thrombin
t. clot test
t. time
thrombocytopenia
t. and absent radius (TAR)
alloimmune t.
immune t.
isoimmune t.
transfusion-induced t.
thrombocytopenic purpura
thromboembolic disease (TE)
thromboembolism
pulmonary t.
venous t.
thrombolytic therapy
thrombophlebitis
deep vein t.
pelvic t.
pelvic vein t.
septic pelvic t.
superficial t.
thromboplastin
thrombosis, pl. **thromboses**
cerebral t.
coronary t.
deep vein t.
deep venous t. (DVT)
maternal cortical vein t.
ovarian vein t.
placental t.
renal vascular t.
venous t.
thrombotic
t. microangiopathy
t. phlegmasia
t. thrombocytopenic purpura (TTP)
thromboxane
t. dominance
thromboxane A_2
thrombus, pl. **thrombi**
thumb retractors
thymectomy
thymic-dependent deficiency
thymic lymphocyte antigen (TL)
thymine
thymosin
thymus gland
Thyro-Block
thyroglobulin
thyrohypophysial syndrome

thyroid
t. autoantibody
t. cancer
t. dysfunction
t. function
t. hormone
t. index
t. neoplasia
t. nodule
t. storm
thyroid-binding globulin (TBG)
thyroidectomy
thyroiditis
Hashimoto's t.
postpartum t.
thyroid-stimulating
t.-s. hormone (TSH)
t.-s. immunoglobulin
Thyrolar
thyrotoxicosis
thyrotrope
thyrotropic hormone
thyrotropin
chorionic t.
thyrotropin-releasing
t.-r. hormone (TRH)
t.-r. hormone stimulation test
thyroxine (T_4)
L-thyroxine
thyroxine-binding
t.-b. globulin
t.-b. protein (TBP)
Thytropar
TIA
transient ischemic attack
Ticar
ticarcillin
Ticon
tidal volume
Tietze's syndrome
Tigan
tilt test
time
activated partial thromboplastin t. (APTT)
bleeding t.
cell generation t.
circulation t.
doubling t.
gastric emptying t.
kaolin clotting t.
Lee-White clotting t.
partial thromboplastin t. (PTT)
t. position scan
prothrombin t.
recovery t.
thrombin t.
Timolide
timolol
Timoptic
Tindal
Tisit
tissue
adipose t.
anechoic t.
attenuating t.
breast biopsy t.
connective t.
echogenic t.
ectopic endometrial t.
fibrous connective t.
t. forceps
glandular t.
granulation t.
intralobular connective t.
lymphoid t.
maternal t.
paravaginal soft t.
perilobular connective t.
placental t.
t. regeneration
residual ductal t.
retroperitoneal soft t.
scar t.
sonolucent t.
splenic t.
t. study
syngeneic t.
t. thromboplastin-inhibition test
t. tolerance
t. transplant
trophoblastic t.
xenogeneic t.
TL
thymic lymphocyte antigen
TNF
tumor necrosis factor
TNM classification
tumor nodal metastasis classification
tobramycin

tococardiography
tocodynagraph
tocodynamometer
tocodynamometry
tocograph
tocography
tocology
tocolysis
tocolytic
t. agent
t. therapy
tocometer
tocophobia
Today
Tofranil
tolazamide
tolazoline hydrochloride
tolbutamide
Tolectin
tolerance
antigen t.
carbohydrate t.
glucose t.
immunologic t.
radiation t.
tolfenamic acid
tolmetin
toluidine
t. blue
t. blue test
tomography
computed t. (CT)
hypocycloidal t.
Tompkins median bivalving technique
tonus
baseline t.
topical
t. iodine application
t. testosterone
t. treatment
TORCH
toxoplasmosis, rubella, cytomegalovirus, and herpes simplex
TORCH syndrome
torsion
adnexal t.
ovarian t.
splenic t.
torticollis
Totacillin
total
t. abdominal hysterectomy (TAH)
t. body water
t. exenteration
t. mastectomy
t. parenteral nutrition (TPN)
t. pelvic exenteration
t. perineal rupture
t. placenta previa
t. pulmonary resistance
t. testosterone index
towel clip
toxemia, toxicemia
preeclamptic t.
t. of pregnancy
toxemic
t. rash of pregnancy
t. retinopathy of pregnancy
toxic
t. megacolon
t. shock
t. shock syndrome (TSS)
t. shock syndrome toxin-1
toxicity
bone marrow t.
toxin
bacterial t.
environmental t.
toxin-1
toxic shock syndrome t.-1
toxoid
tetanus t.
Toxoplasma gondii
toxoplasmosis
congenital t.
fetal t.
toxoplasmosis, rubella, cytomegalovirus, and herpes simplex (TORCH)
TPI
Treponema pallidum immobilization
TPN
total parenteral nutrition
trace metal
tracheal intubation
trachelectomy
trachelitis
trachelobregmatic diameter
trachelopanus
trachelopexia, trachelopexy

tracheloplasty
trachelorrhaphy
trachelotomy
tracheoesophageal fistula
trachoma
tract
gastrointestinal t.
genital t.
intestinal t.
reproductive t.
respiratory t.
urinary t.
traction
t. atrophy
axis t.
trait
autosomal dominant t.
autosomal recessive t.
mendelian t.
sickle cell t.
threshold t.
X-linked t.
Trandate
tranexamic acid
tranquilizer
transabdominal
t. cervicoisthmic cerclage
t. chorionic villus sampling
transaminase
serum t.
transanimation
transcapillary
transcatheter embolization
transcervical
t. balloon tuboplasty
t. chorionic villus sampling
t. division
t. endometrial resection
t. resection
transcortin
transcriptase
reverse t.
transcription
transcutaneous measurement
transdermal
t. administration
t. hormone replacement therapy
t. medication patch
transducer
transfer
embryo t.
t. factor
gamete intrafallopian t. (GIFT)
gas t.
linear energy t. (LET)
placental t.
pronuclear stage tubal t. (PROST)
t. RNA (tRNA)
tubal embryo t. (TET)
tubal embryo stage t. (TEST)
in vitro fertilization/embryo t. (IVF/ET)
zygote intrafallopian t. (ZIFT)
transferrin
transformation
t. zone
transforming
t. growth factor
t. growth factor alpha (TGFα)
t. growth factor beta (TGFβ)
transfusion
autologous t.
blood t.
t. controversy
erythrocyte t.
fetal t.
intraperitoneal blood t.
intraperitoneal fetal t.
intrauterine t.
intrauterine intraperitoneal fetal t.
intravascular t.
leukocyte t.
massive t.
percutaneous fetal t.
placental t.
platelet t.
prophylactic red-cell t.
twin-twin t.
umbilical cord t.
transfusion-induced thrombocytopenia
transient
t. congenital hypothyroidism
t. fetal distress
t. ischemic attack (TIA)
t. tachypnea
transillumination

transition
fetal-neonatal t.
translation
translocation
balanced t.
t. carrier
chromosomal t.
reciprocal t.
robertsonian t.
unbalanced t.
transmigration
ovular t.
transmission
maternal-fetal t.
t. medium
perinatal t.
pressure t.
sexual t.
viral t.
transperineal implant
transperitoneal cesarean section
transplacental
t. hemorrhage
t. passage
transplant
liver t.
organ t.
tissue t.
transplantation
t. antigen
bone marrow t.
t. immunology
kidney t.
liver t.
organ t.
pituitary gland t.
renal t.
transport
t. disorder
egg t.
transposed adnexa
transposition
t. of great vessel
t. of ovary
transrectal
t. approach
transsexual
transsphenoidal
t. microsurgical resection
t. operation
transurethral
t. electrocautery
t. marsupialization
transvaginal
t. cone
t. implant
t. sonography
t. transducer probe
t. ultrasound
transverse
t. cervical ligament
t. diameter
t. fundal incision of Strassmann
t. lie
occiput t. (OT)
t. oval pelvis
t. presentation
t. ridge
t. scan
t. vaginal septum
tranylcypromine
trapped ovum
Trasicor
trauma, pl. **traumata, traumas**
birth t.
blunt t.
childhood genital t.
fetal t.
genital tract t.
maternal t.
psychological t.
traumatic
t. amenorrhea
t. injury
t. vaginitis
Travamine
trazodone
treatment
aggressive t.
antenatal phenobarbitol t.
compelled medical t.
continuous/combined t.
exchange transfusion t.
hormonal t.
infertility t.
laser t.
prenatal t.
topical t.
transrectal surgical t.
ureteral surgical t.
treatment-associated pregnancy
treatment-independent pregnancy
Trecator-SC
Trental

Treponema
Treponema pallidum immobilization (TPI)
Treponema pallidum
tretinoin
Trexan
TRH
thyrotropin-releasing hormone
triacetyloleandomycin
trial
chemotherapy phase t.
t. forceps
labor t.
triamcinolone acetonide
triamterene
triangle
Hesselbach's t.
triangular
t. ligament
t. uterus
Triasox
Triazole
Trichlorex
trichlormethiazide
trichloroacetic acid
trichloroethylene
2,4,5-trichlorophenoxyacetic acid
Trichomonas
Trichomonas infection
Trichomonas species
Trichomonas vaginalis
Trichomonas vaginalis vaginitis
trichomoniasis
t. vaginitis
trichorhinophalangeal syndrome
tricyclic antidepressant
tridihexethyl chloride
Tridione
tridymus
triethylenethiophosphoramide
trifluoperazine hydrochloride
triflupromazine hydrochloride
trigger point
triglyceride
trigone
trigonitis
Trihexane
Trihexy
trihexyphenidyl
triiodothyronine (T_3)
reverse t.
Trikacide
Trilafon
Tri-Levlen 5/
Tri-Levlen 6/
Tri-Levlen 10/
trimeprazine
trimester
first t.
second t.
third t.
trimethadione
trimethaphan camsylate
trimethobenzamide hydrochloride
trimethoprim
trimethoprim-sulfamethoxazole (SMZ-TMP)
trimipramine
Trimox
Trimpex
Trimstat
Trimtabs
Tri-Norinyl 5/
Tri-Norinyl 7/
Tri-Norinyl 9/
triodurin
triosephosphate isomerase
tripelennamine hydrochloride
Triphasil 5/
Triphasil 6/
Triphasil 10/
triphosphate
adenosine t. (ATP)
5′-triphosphate
guanosine -t. (GTP)
Triple
T. bromide
triplet
triple X syndrome
triploid fetus
triploidy
triprolidine hydrochloride
Triptil
trisomy
autosomal t.
trisomy 13
trisomy 15
trisomy 16
trisomy 18
trisomy 21
trisphosphate
inositol t.
tRNA
transfer RNA
transfer ribonucleic acid

Trobicin
troleandomycin
trophoblast
t. sampling
trophoblastic
t. cell
t. disease
t. embolus
t. neoplasia
t. pseudotumor
t. tissue
t. tumor
trophospongia
trophotropism
tropical bubo
tropic hormone
troponin
trousers
antishock t.
true
t. conjugate
t. hermaphroditism
t. incontinence
t. knot
t. knot of umbilical cord
t. labor
t. precocious puberty
t. uterine inertia
Trymegen
tryptophan
TSH
thyroid-stimulating hormone
T-shaped
T.-s. constriction ring
T.-s. uterus
TSS
toxic shock syndrome
TTP
thrombotic thrombocytopenic purpura
tubage
tubal
t. abortion
t. colic
t. diverticulum
t. dysmenorrhea
t. embryo stage transfer (TEST)
t. embryo transfer (TET)
t. endometriosis
t. endometrium
t. factor
t. gestation
t. insufflation
t. ligation
t. ligation band technique
t. mass
t. metaplasia
t. microsurgery
t. obstruction
t. pregnancy
t. reconstruction
t. ring
t. rupture
t. sterilization
tube
Cantor t.
endotracheal t.
fallopian t.
Miller-Abbott t.
nasogastric t.
neural t.
pus t.
uterine t.
tubectomy
tubercle
genital t.
Montgomery's t.'s
Morgagni's t.
Müller's t.
Rokitansky t.
tuberculosis
endometrial t.
pulmonary t.
tuberculous salpingitis
tuberous
t. mole
t. subchorial hematoma of the decidua
tuboabdominal pregnancy
tubocornual
t. microsurgery
t. reanastomosis
tuboendometrial cell
tubo-ovarian
t.-o. abscess
t.-o. complex
t.-o. pregnancy
t.-o. varicocele
tubo-ovariectomy
tubo-ovaritis
tuboplasty
transcervical balloon t.
tubotorsion, tubatorsion

tubouterine
t. implantation
t. pregnancy
tubular carcinoma
tubule
annular t.
mesonephric t.
seminiferous t.
tubulointerstitial disease
Tucker-McLean
T.-M. forceps
Tucker-McLean-Luikhart forceps
tularemia
tumor
adenomatoid t.
adenomatoid oviduct t.
adnexal t.
adrenal t.
adrenal rest t.
androgen-producing t.
t. angiogenesis factor (TAF)
angiomatoid t.
t. antigen
t. antigenicity
t. ascites
autochthonous t.
benign t.
bladder t.
bone t.
borderline epithelial ovarian t.
borderline ovarian t.
Brenner t.
t. burden
carcinoid t.
central nervous system t.
cervical stump t.
colorectal t.
endodermal sinus t.
endometrioid t.
epithelial t.
epithelial stromal t.
genital tract t.
germ cell t.
gestational trophoblastic t.
gonadal stromal ovarian t.
granulosa cell t.
granulosa-stromal cell t.
hilar cell t.
t. immunology
t. immunotherapy
intracranial t.
Krukenberg's t.
Leydig cell t.
lipid cell t.
lipid cell ovarian t.
lipoid ovarian t.
liver t.
malignant t.
malignant mixed müllerian t. (MMMT)
t. marker
t. mass
mesonephroid t.
mixed germ cell t.
mixed mesodermal t.
mixed uterine t.
monodermal t.
mucinous t.
t. necrosis factor (TNF)
t. necrosis factor-α
t. nodal metastasis classification (TNM classification)
ovarian t.
parovarian t.
t. persistence
persistent trophoblastic t.
pituitary gland t.
pregnancy t.
t. progression
Recklinghausen's t.
t. regression
serous t.
Sertoli cell t.
Sertoli-Leydig cell t.
sex cord-stromal t.
sex cord-stromal germ cell t.
t. size
trophoblastic t.
ulcerative t.
uterine corpus t.
virilizing t.
Wilms' t.
yolk sac t.
tumor-associated antigen (TAA)
tumor-cloning assay
tumor-limiting factor
tumorous hyperprolactinemia
tumor-specific transplantation antigen
tungsten target
tunica
t. albuginea
Turner's syndrome

turnover
bone t.
turtle sign
Tusstat
twilight sleep
twin
allantoidoangiopagous t.'s
t. birth
conjoined t.'s
t. delivery
t. gestation
growth-discordant t.
locked t.
membranous t.
monozygotic t.'s
omphaloangiopagous t.'s
t. placenta
t. pregnancy
second t.
twinning
twin-twin transfusion
two-cell
t.-c. mechanism
t.-c. zygote
two-tail test
Tylenol
Tylox
tympanites
uterine t.
type
t. I diabetes
t. I dip
t. II diabetes
t. II dip
t. II pneumonocyte
t. 16 *Papillomavirus*
typhoid
t. autoantibody
t. fever
t. vaccine
tyropanoate sodium
tyrosine
t. kinase

GOT A GOOD WORD FOR THE NEXT EDITION OF

THIS STEDMAN'S WORD BOOK?

Help us keep future editions of this **Stedman's Word Book** fresh and up-to-date with new words and new ideas!

What's going on in your field? Are there new terms being used in this specialty? Are there better, easier ways for organizing the book's content?

Be specific! We want to know how we can make this **Stedman's Word Book** the very best specialty medical word reference possible for you. So go ahead and fill-in the lines below with your best thoughts and recommendations. Attach a separate sheet of paper if you have to—*you* are our most important contributor and we want to know what's on *your* mind!

Thanks!

(PLEASE TYPE OR PRINT CLEARLY)

OK, here's what I think: ______________________________

____

____

____

____

____

____

____

____

____

All done? Great, just detach this card and mail today. No postage necessary, and thanks again!

Name ______________________________ Title ____________

Facility ______________________ ______________________

Address ____

____

City ____________________ State ________ Zip _____-_____

Day Telephone No. (   ) ____________________

Williams & Wilkins
428 East Preston Street • Baltimore, MD 21202-6564

7942-5 OB-GYN

NO POSTAGE
NECESSARY
IF MAILED
IN THE
UNITED STATES

BUSINESS REPLY MAIL

FIRST CLASS PERMIT NO. 724 BALTIMORE, MD

POSTAGE WILL BE PAID BY ADDRESSEE

Williams & Wilkins
ATTN: REFERENCE DIVISION/Gail Russell
P.O.Box Box 1496
Baltimore, Maryland 21298-9724

U

UDI
urinary diagnostic index
UICC
International Union Against Cancer
ulcer
genital u.
Lipschütz' u.
peptic u.
rectal postradiation u.
vaginal u.
ulcerative
u. colitis
u. tumor
ulcus, pl. **ulcera**
u. vulvae acutum
Ultracef
ultrasonography
Doppler u.
gray-scale u.
ultrasound, ultrasonic
A-mode u.
antenatal u.
u. assessment
B-mode u.
u. cephalometry
u. diagnosis
Doppler u.
duplex u.
u. egg recovery
fetal u.
u. fetometry
u. guidance
M-mode u.
prenatal u.
real-time u.
u. surveillance
transvaginal u.
vaginal u.
u. visualization
umbilical
u. artery
u. artery flow velocity waveform
u. blood flow
u. blood sampling
u. circulation
u. cord
u. cord transfusion
u. cyst
u. fistula
u. fungus
u. hernia
u. ligament
u. souffle
u. vein
umbilicus
umbrella
vascular u.
unavoidable hemorrhage
unbalanced translocation
undernourishment
maternal u.
undifferentiated
u. carcinoma of ovary
u. gonad
unexplained infertility
unicolic uterus
unicornous, unicorn, pl. **uteri**
unicornous uterus
unicornuate uterus
unilateral salpingo-oophorectomy
uninterrupted estrogen
Unipen
unit
fetal-placental u.
high-risk pregnancy u.
maternal-placental u.
maternal-placental-fetal u.
pilosebaceous u.
terminal duct lobular u. (TDLU)
Unitensen
universal joint syndrome
unopposed estrogen
unresponsiveness
immunologic u.
unruptured
u. ectopic pregnancy
u. tubal gestation
u. tubal pregnancy
unsaturated fat
unstable lie
u-PA
urokinase-type plasminogen activator
uptake
minute oxygen u.
Uracel

urachal
u. cyst
u. fistula
urachus
urate clearance
Urban's operation
urea
u. clearance
Ureaphil
Ureaplasma urealyticum
Urecholine
uremia
ureter
double u.
ectopic u.
ureteral, ureteric
u. dysmenorrhea
u. fistulae
u. node
u. obstruction
ureterocervical
ureteroneocystostomy
ureterotubal anastomosis
ureteroureteral anastomosis
ureterouterine
ureterovaginal
u. fistula
urethra
penile u.
urethral
u. angle
u. caruncle
u. closure pressure profile
u. diverticulum
u. function
u. gland
u. opening
u. pressure
u. prolapse
u. spasm
u. sphincter
u. syndrome
urethritis
anterior u.
follicular u.
granular u.
nonspecific u.
u. petrificans
posterior u.
simple u.
specific u.
u. venerea
urethrocele
urethrocystometry
urethrography
urethropexy
retropubic u.
urethroscopy
urethrovaginal fistula
urethrovesical angle
Urex
urge incontinence
urgency
urinary u.
uric
u. acid
Uridon
urinalysis
urinary
u. bladder
u. calculus
u. concentrating capacity
u. conduit
u. diagnostic index (UDI)
u. diversion
u. exertional incontinence
u. fistula
u. frequency
u. incontinence
u. sediment
u. stent
u. stress incontinence
u. system
u. tract
u. tract
u. tract infection
u. tract obstruction
u. urgency
urination
fetal u.
urine
u. concentration test
u. culture
u. flow
u. output
residual u.
u. test
Urispas
urodynamic study
urogenital
u. diaphragm
u. fistula
u. fold
u. sinus
u. structure
urokinase

urokinase-type plasminogen activator (u-PA)
Urolene Blue
urolithiasis
urologic, urological
u. evaluation
u. history
u. injury
urology
uropathy
bilateral u.
fetal u.
obstructive u.
Urozide
urticarial papule
use
conservative drug u.
early drug u.
illicit drug u.
maternal aspirin u.
maternal cocaine u.
oral contraceptive u.
prophylactic aspirin u.
uterectomy
uteri
corpus u.
myomata u.
uterine
u. abnormality
u. absence
u. access
u. action
u. activity
u. anomaly
u. artery
u. atony
u. bleeding
u. blood flow
u. calculus
u. colic
u. compression
u. constriction ring
u. contraction
u. corpus
u. cramping
u. decompression
u. dysmenorrhea
u. endolymphatic stroma
u. endometrial stroma
u. epithelial stroma
u. epithelium
u. evaluation
u. factor
u. fibroid
u. fundal height
u. gland
u. hematoma
u. hemostasis
u. hernia syndrome
u. horn
u. incision
u. inertia
u. infection
u. insufficiency
u. malposition
u. mass
u. massage
u. milk
u. myometrium
u. necrosis
u. pathology
u. perforation
u. pregnancy
u. prolapse
u. quiescence
u. relaxation
u. retroflexion
u. retroversion
u. rupture
u. sacculation
u. scar separation
u. screening
u. segment
u. septa
u. sinus
u. sinusoid
u. size
u. souffle
u. sound
u. suspension
u. tube
u. tympanites
u. vein
u. vessel
uterine-placental perfusion
uterismus
uteritis
in utero
uteroabdominal pregnancy
uterocystostomy
uterofixation
uterolith
uterometer
utero-ovarian
u.-o. ligament
u.-o. varicocele

uteroperitoneal fistula
uteropexy
uteroplacental
- u. apoplexy
- u. blood flow
- u. insufficiency
- u. perfusion
- u. sinus
- u. vessel

uteroplasty
uterosacral ligament
uterosalpingography
uteroscope
uteroscopy
uterotomy
uterotonic
uterotonin
uterotropin
uterotubography
uterovaginal canal
uterus, pl. **uteri**
- u. acollis
- anomalous u.
- arcuate u., u. arcuatus
- u. bicameratus vetularum
- bicornate u., u. bicornis
- bifid u., u. bifidus
- biforate u., u. biforis
- u. bilocularis
- bipartite u., u. bipartitus
- capped u.
- communicating u.
- cordiform u., u. cordiformis
- Couvelaire u.
- didelphic u.
- u. didelphys
- double-mouthed u.
- duplex u., u. duplex
- fibromyoma of u.
- gravid u.
- heart-shaped u.
- incudiform u., u. incudiformis
- intramural myoma of u.
- large-for-dates u.
- one-horned u.
- u. parvicollis
- ruptured u.
- septate u., u. septus
- subseptate u., u. subseptus
- symmetric communicating u.
- triangular u., u. triangularis
- T-shaped u.
- unicolic u.
- unicorn u., u. unicornis
- unicornuate u.

utricle
- prostatic u.

V

Vabra
V. aspirator
V. suction
VAC
vincristine, actinomycin D, cyclophosphamide
vaccination
vaccine
Bacille bilié de Calmette-Guérin v.
bacillus Calmette-Guérin v.
BCG v.
cholera v.
Escherichia coli v.
hepatitis B v.
inactivated poliovirus v.
influenza v.
live poliovirus v.
live-virus v.
measles v.
meningococcal polysaccharide v.
Meningococcus v.
mumps v.
Pasteur Institute bacillus Calmette-Guérin v.
plague v.
pneumococcal v.
polyvalent pneumococcal v.
rabies v.
rubella v.
Sabin v.
Salk v.
smallpox v.
tularemia v.
typhoid v.
yellow fever v.
VACTERL syndrome
vacuole
vacuolization
vacuum
v. aspiration
v. aspirator
v. extraction
v. extractor
vagina
vaginal
v. absence
v. adenocarcinoma
v. adenosis
v. administration
v. agenesis
v. anomaly
v. antibiotic cream
v. artery
v. atresia
v. atrophy
v. bleeding
v. cancer
v. candidiasis
v. carcinoma
v. celiotomy
v. contraceptive
v. cyst
v. cystourethropexy
v. cytology
v. delivery
v. dilator
v. discharge
v. douching
v. dysmenorrhea
v. dysontogenetic cyst
v. ectopic anus
v. embryonic cyst
v. epithelial abnormality
v. estrogen therapy
v. examination
v. GIFT
v. hematoma
v. hood
v. hysterectomy
v. hysterotomy
v. inclusion cyst
v. infection
v. injury
v. intraepithelial neoplasia (VAIN)
v. laceration
v. lithotomy
v. lubricant
v. microflora
v. mucosa
v. myomectomy
v. opening
operative obstetrics
v. outlet
v. perineorrhaphy
v. pH
v. plate
v. pool

vaginal *(continued)*
v. prolapse
v. repair
v. ring contraception
v. secretion
v. sonography
v. sponge
v. squamous metaplasia
v. stump prolapse
v. suppository
v. surgery
v. tampon
v. terminus
v. tumor
v. ulcer
v. ultrasound
v. vault
v. vault prolapse
v. venous plexus
v. wall repair
v. yeast
vaginalis
portio v.
vaginapexy
vaginectomy
vaginism
vaginismus
posterior v.
vaginitis, pl. **vaginitides**
adhesive v., v. adhesiva
amebic v.
atrophic v.
Candida v.
chlamydial v.
v. cystica
desquamative inflammatory v.
v. emphysematosa
monilial v.
nonspecific v.
pinworm v.
recurrent v.
senile v., v. senilis
streptococcal v.
traumatic v.
Trichomonas vaginalis v.
vaginocele
vaginodynia
vaginofixation
vaginohysterectomy
vaginomycosis
vaginopathy
vaginoperineoplasty
vaginoperineorraphy
vaginoperineotomy
vaginopexy
vaginoplasty
vaginoscopy
pediatric v.
vaginosis
bacterial v.
mycotic v.
vaginotomy
vagitus uterinus
VAIN
vaginal intraepithelial neoplasia
Valadol
valerate
betamethasone v.
estradiol v.
Valergen
validity
Valisone
Valium
Valorin
Valpin 50
valproate
sodium v.
valproic acid
value
acid-base v.
complement v.
fetal blood v.
maturation v.
P v.
valve
valvotomy
valvular
v. heart disease
v. prosthesis
Vancenase
Vancenase AQ
Vanceril
Vancocin
vancomycin
vanishing
v. testes syndrome
v. twin syndrome
Vanquin
Vapo-Iso
Vaponefrin
vaporization
variability
baseline v. of fetal heart rate
beat-to-beat v.

fetal heart rate v.
interpretation v.
variable deceleration
variation
beat-to-beat v. of fetal heart rate
coefficient of v. (CV)
interobserver v.
observer v.
varicella
varicella-zoster
v.-z. immune globulin
v.-z. virus
varicocele
ovarian v.
tubo-ovarian v.
utero-ovarian v.
varicocelectomy
varicomphalus
varicosity
varix, pl. **varices**
esophageal varices
gelatinous v.
vulvar v.
vas, gen. **vasis**, gen. and pl. **vasorum**, pl. **vasa**
vasal
vascular
v. anomaly
v. calcification
v. channel
v. communication
v. complication
v. disease
v. engorgement
v. headache
v. injury
v. leiomyoma
v. metastasis
v. reactivity
v. resistance
v. spider
v. umbrella
vascularization
chorionic v.
vasculitis
rheumatoid v.
vas deferens
vasectomy
vasitis
vasoactive intestinal peptide (VIP)
vasocongestion
Vasodilan
vasomotor symptom
vasopressin
arginine v.
vasopressor
vasorum
Vasospan
vasospasm
Vasotec
vasotocin
arginine v.
Vasoxyl
vault
vaginal v.
VBP
vinblastine, bleomycin, cisplatin
V-Cillin K
VC-K
VDRL
Venereal Disease Research Laboratories
vectis
Veetids
vegan
vegetarian
v. diet
Veillonella
vein
dilated collateral v.
iliac v.
maternal cortical v.
ovarian v.
umbilical v.
uterine v.
velamen, pl. **velamina**
v. vulvae
Velban
vellus hair
velocimetry
Doppler v.
velocity
v. flow profile
Velosef
Veltane
velum, pl. **vela**
vena
v. cava
v. caval filter
v. caval interruption
Venereal
V. Disease Research Laboratories (VDRL)
venereal
v. bubo

venereal *(continued)*
v. disease
v. lymphogranuloma
v. wart
venereology
venography
radionuclide v.
venous
v. collateral
v. oozing
v. thromboembolism
v. thrombosis
venter
v. propendens
ventilation
v. by mask
v. scintigraphy
ventilation/perfusion (V/Q)
Ventolin
ventouse
ventral hernia
ventricular
v. function
v. response rate
v. septal defect
v. tachycardia
ventriculomegaly
ventriculoperitoneal shunt
Veralba
verapamil
***Veratrum* alkaloid**
vergeture
Veriloid
Vermox
vernix
verrucous carcinoma
version
bimanual v.
bipolar v.
Braxton-Hicks v.
cephalic v.
combined v.
external v.
internal v.
pelvic v.
podalic v.
postural v.
Potter's v.
spontaneous v.
Wright's v.
vertebral
v. artery
v. bone loss
v. bone mass
v. compression fracture
vertex, pl. **vertices**
v. presentation
vertical hymen
vertically
v. acquired infection
very-low-birth-weight infant
very low-density lipoprotein (VLDL)
vesicle
chorionic v.
germinal v.
vesicocele
vesicofixation
vesicouterine fistula
vesicovaginal
v. fistula
v. repair
vesicovaginorectal
v. fistula
vesicular mole
vessel
chorioallantoic v.
corkscrew v.
great v.
hairpin v.
v. spread
transposition of great v.'s
uterine v.
uteroplacental v.
vestibular
v. adenitis
v. anus
v. bulb
v. cyst
v. duct
v. gland
vestibule
vestibulitis
vulvar v.
viability
fetal v.
viable
Vibramycin
vibroacoustic stimulation
vicarious menstruation
Vicryl
V. suture
vidarabine
view
axillary v.
colposcopic v.

craniocaudal v.
exaggerated craniocaudal v.
four-chamber v.
lateral oblique v.
lateromedial oblique v.
long-axis v.
medial oblique v.
mediolateral v.
pulmonary artery/ductus v.
short-axis v.
spot compression v.

villositis

villous
v. artery
v. placenta

villus, pl. **villi**
chorionic villi
placental v.

VIN
vulvar intraepithelial neoplasia

vinblastine

vinblastine, bleomycin, cisplatin (VBP)

***Vinca* alkaloid**

vincristine

vincristine, actinomycin D, cyclophosphamide (VAC)

VIN III
vulvar carcinoma in situ

violet
crystal v.
gentian v.

VIP
vasoactive intestinal peptide

viprynium

Vira-A

viral
v. infection
v. pneumonitis
v. transmission

Virazole

Virchow
pneumonia alba of V.

virgin

virginal
v. breast hypertrophy

virginity

virilescence

virilism
adrenal v.

virilization

virilizing
v. adenoma
v. 3α-androstanediol glucuronide
v. tumor

virion
intranuclear v.

virulent bubo

virus
acquired immunodeficiency syndrome-related v. (ARV)
hepatitis A v.
hepatitis B v.
herpes simplex v. (HSV)
horizontal transmission of v.
human immunodeficiency v. (HIV)
human papilloma v. (HPV)
human T-cell leukemia v. (HTLV)
human T-cell leukemia v. type III (HTLV-III)
influenza v.
lymphadenopathy-associated v. (LAV)
mumps v.
rubella v.
varicella-zoster v.

visceral peritoneum

Visken

Vistaril

visual
v. change
v. disturbance
v. field

visualization

Vitabee 6

vital
v. capacity
v. sign

vitamin
v. A
v. B_6
v. B_{12}
v. B complex
B complex v.'s
v. C
v. D
v. D-binding protein
v. D-resistant rickets
v. E
v. K prophylaxis
v. metabolism

vitamin *(continued)*
- v. requirement
- v. supplement

Vita Plus E
vitelline
- v. cord
- v. fistula
- v. membrane

vitellointestinal cyst
in vitro fertilization
in vitro fertilization/embryo transfer (IVF/ET)
Vivactil
viviparity
viviparous
in vivo fertilization
Vivol
VLDL
- very low-density lipoprotein

voiding
voiding dysfunction
volatile
- v. acid
- v. anesthetic

volt
- electron-v. (eV, ev)

volume
- blood v.
- closing v.
- v. expansion
- fetal blood v.
- v. flow
- forced expiratory v.
- intrauterine v.
- lung v.
- minute ventilatory v.
- plasma v.
- red cell v.
- residual v.
- semen v.
- tidal v.

voluntary sterilization
volvulus
vomiting
- nausea and v.
- v. of pregnancy

VP-16
V/Q
- ventilation/perfusion
  - V/Q mismatch
  - V/Q scan

vulgaris
- acne v.

vulva
vulvar
- v. atypia
- v. biopsy
- v. cancer staging
- v. carcinoma
- v. carcinoma in situ (VIN III)
- v. dystrophy
- v. inclusion cyst
- v. infection
- v. intraepithelial neoplasia (VIN)
- v. malignancy
- v. varix
- v. vestibule
- v. vestibulitis

vulvectomy
- radical v.
- simple v.
- skinning v.

vulvismus
vulvitis
- adhesive v.
- chronic atrophic v.
- chronic hypertrophic v.
- follicular v.
- leukoplakic v.

vulvodynia
vulvovaginal
- v. anus
- v. candidiasis
- v. carcinoma
- v. cystectomy
- v. lesion
- v. outlet

vulvovaginitis
- premenarchal v.

Vytone

W

Wade
Roe v. W.
Wagenstein needle holder
waist:hip ratio
Walcher position
Waldeyer
germinal epithelium of W.
W.'s fossae
Walker's chart
wall
abdominal w.
opposing w.
Walthard's cell rest
Walther's dilator
Walton report
warfarin
warfarin embryopathy
Warfilone
wart
anogenital w.
flat w.
genital w.
venereal w.
water w.
washed
w. intrauterine insemination
w. spermatozoa
wastage
early pregnancy w.
fetal w.
pregnancy w.
reproductive w.
wasting
salt w.
water
w. excretion
w. intoxication
w. loss
w. metabolism
total body w.
w. wart
waters
bag of w.
false w.
Waters' operation
waveform
arterial w.
discordant artery flow velocity w.
Doppler w.
flow velocity w.
wean
weaning
Webster's operation
wedge resection
Wegener's granulomatosis
Wehamine
Wehdryl
Wehless
weight
birth w.
body w.
fetal w.
w. gain
w. loss
low birth w.
maternal w.
placental w.
w. reduction
very low birth w.
weight-bearing bone
weighted speculum
Weightrol
well-being
fetal w.-b.
well-born
right to be w.-b.
well-circumscribed carcinoma
Wellcovorin
well-defined mass
Wells v. Ortho Pharmaceutical
Wertheim's operation
Western blot
West's syndrome
wet
w. mount
w. smear
Wharton's jelly
whiff test
white
w. blood cell
w. epithelium
w. infarct
w. leg
WHO
whole-abdomen irradiation
whole blood
whole-pelvis irradiation
wide plane

Wigand maneuver
Willett's
  W. clamp
  W. forceps
Wilms' tumor
Wilpowr
Wilson-Mikity syndrome
Wilson's disease
window
  therapeutic w.
wire
  iridium w.
witch's milk
withdrawal
  w. bleeding
  estrogen w.
witness
  expert w.
Wolfe classification of breast cancer
wolffian
  w. duct
  w. rest
Wolff-Parkinson-White syndrome
Wolfram's syndrome
Wolman's disease
woman
  androgenized w.
  battered w.
  euprolactinemic w.
  hirsute w.
  hypoestrogenic w.
  hypogonadal w.
  infertile w.
  lactating w.
  normotensive w.
  perimenopausal w.
  postmenopausal w.
  pregnant w.
womb
  falling of the w.
  scarred w.
Woods' screw maneuver
Word bladder catheter
work environment
wound
  abdominal w.
  w. breakdown
  gunshot w.
  w. infection
  stab w.
Wright's
  W. stain
  W. version
wrongful
  w. birth and life
  w. conception
Wyamycin-S
Wycillin
Wygesic
Wymox
Wytensin

X

χ^2
chi-square
X
X. chromosome
X. isochromosome
45,X
45,X karyotype
45,X syndrome
Xanax
xanthine
X-chromosome abnormality
xenogeneic tissue
xenograft
xeroderma pigmentosum
xeromammography
xeromenia
xerotocia
X-linked
X.-l. disorder
X.-l. gene
X.-l. trait
XO
45,XO
X-Prep
x-ray
x.-r. pelvimetry
x.-r. therapy
XX
X. chromosome
X. hermaphroditism
X. male syndrome
46,XX
46,XX karyotype
46,XX male
XXX
47,XXX
47,XXX syndrome
47,XXY
47,XXY karyotype
47,XXY syndrome
69,XXY
46,XY
46,XY karyotype
XY gonadal dysgenesis
Xylocaine
XYY syndrome

Y

Y
Y. chromosome
Y. chromosome-specific DNA sequence
year
postnatal y.
10-year surveillance
yeast
y. infection
vaginal y.
yellow fever vaccine
Yodoxin
yolk
y. sac
Y-specific
Y.-s. DNA
Yutapar
YY
YY syndrome

Z

Zantac
Zarontin
Zaroxolyn
ZDV
zidovudine
Zetran
zidovudine (ZDV)
ZIFT
zygote intrafallopian transfer
zinc
z. oxide
z. peroxide
Z-line
zomepirac sodium
zona
z. basalis
z. compacta
z. functionalis
z. pellucida
z. reaction
z. spongiosa
zona-free
z.-f. hamster egg penetration test
zonary placenta
Zondek-Aschheim test
zone
Barnes' z.
cervical z.
cervical transformation z.
normal transformation z.
transformation z.
zoogonous
zoogony
Zoon's erythroplasia
zoster immune globulin
Zovirax
zuclopenthixol
zygosity
zygote
z. intrafallopian transfer (ZIFT)
two-cell z.
zygotene stage

Appendix 1
Cesarean Delivery

Adson forceps
Adson pick-ups
Allis clamp
Army-Navy retractor
Babcock clamp
Balfour retractor
bandage scissors
Billroth tumor forceps
bladder retractor
clamp
Crile-Wood needle holder
curved hemostat
DeLee universal retractor
forceps
Heaney-Ballentine forceps
Heaney needle holder
hemostat
holder
Kelly clamp
Kocher clamp
Lister scissors
malleable retractor
Mayo curved scissors
Mayo-Hegar needle holder
Mayo straight scissors
Metzenbaum long scissors
Metzenbaum scissors
Murless head retractor
Ochsner forceps
O'Sullivan-O'Connor retractor
Pennington clamp
Phaneuf uterine artery forceps
pick-up
rat tooth pick-ups
retractor
Richardson retractor
Roch-Péan forceps
Schroeder tenaculum forceps
Schroeder vulsella forceps
scissors
Singley forceps
sponge forceps
thumb retractors
tissue forceps

Appendix 2
Dilation and Curettage (D & C)

Auvard speculum
Backhaus clamp
Bozeman uterine dressing forceps
Braun-Schroeder single-tooth tenaculum
clamp
clip
Crile forceps
Crile hemostat
curet
curette
Deaver retractor
dilator
dressing forceps
Duncan's curette
forceps
Graves bivalve speculum
Green uterine curette
Heaney curette
hemostat
holder
Jackson right angle retractor
Jacobs tenaculum
Kelly clamp
Kelly-Gray curette
Kevorkian-Younge biopsy forceps
Kevorkian-Younge curette
Laufe polyp forceps
Mayo-Hegar needle holder
Mayo scissors
Pratt dilator
Randall stone forceps
retractor
Roch-Péan forceps
Schroeder uterine tenaculum
Schubert uterine biopsy forceps
scissors
Sims curette
sound
speculum
sponge forceps
sponge sticks
stick
tenaculum
Thomas curette
Thomas-Gaylor biopsy forceps
tissue forceps
towel clip
towel clip
uterine sound
weighted speculum

Appendix 3
Total Abdominal Hysterectomy

Adson ganglion scissors
Allis clamp
Allis forceps
Army-Navy retractor
Babcock clamp
Balfour bladder blade
Balfour retractor
Ballentine clamp
Billroth tumor forceps
blade
clamp
Deaver retractor
DeBakey clamp
DeBakey tissue forceps
double-tooth tenaculum
dressing forceps
forceps
Goulet retractor
Harrington retractor
Heaney-Ballentine forceps
Heaney clamp
Heaney-Hyst forceps
Heaney needle holder
holder
Jacobs tenaculum
Jorgenson scissors
Kelly clamp
Kocher clamp
Mayo scissors
Ochsner forceps
O'Sullivan-O'Connor retractor
Péan forceps
pedicle clamp
retractor
right angle scissors
Roberts thumb retractor
Roch-Ochs forceps
Russian tissue forceps
Schroeder tenaculum
Schroeder tenaculum forceps
Schroeder vulsella forceps
scissors
single-tooth tenaculum
sponge forceps
sponge holding forceps
tenaculum
thoracic clamp
tissue forceps
Wagenstein needle holder

Appendix 4
Vaginal Delivery

Allis clamp
amniohook
Auvard speculum
Backhaus clamp
Barton's forceps
Baumberger forceps
Billroth tumor forceps
Bill traction handle forceps
Bird's vacuum extractor
Braun episiotomy scissors
clamp
clip
Crile forceps
DeLee forceps
DeWees forceps
Dewey forceps
dressing forceps
Elliot forceps
English lock
extractor
forceps
French lock
Gelpi perineal retractor
German lock
Haig-Fergusson forceps
Halsted mosquito forceps
Hawk-Dennen forceps
Heaney-Ballentine forceps
Heaney needle holder
Hodge's forceps
holder
Kelly clamp
Kelly retractor
Kjelland-Barton forceps
Kjelland-Luikart forceps
Kjelland's forceps
Kobayashi vacuum extractor
lock
Luikart forceps
Malmström vacuum extractor
Mayo-Hegar needle holder
Mayo scissors
McLean forceps
Mityvac vacuum extractor
Murless head extractor
Naegele forceps
Ochsner forceps
Piper's forceps
pivot lock
retractor
Russian tissue forceps
Schroeder tenaculum
scissors
Shute forceps
Silastic cup extractor
Simpson's forceps
sliding lock
speculum
sponge sticks
stick
straight scissors
Tarnier's axis-traction forceps
tenaculum
tissue forceps
towel clip
towel clip
Tucker-McLean-Luikhart forceps

Appendix 5
Fetal Presentations

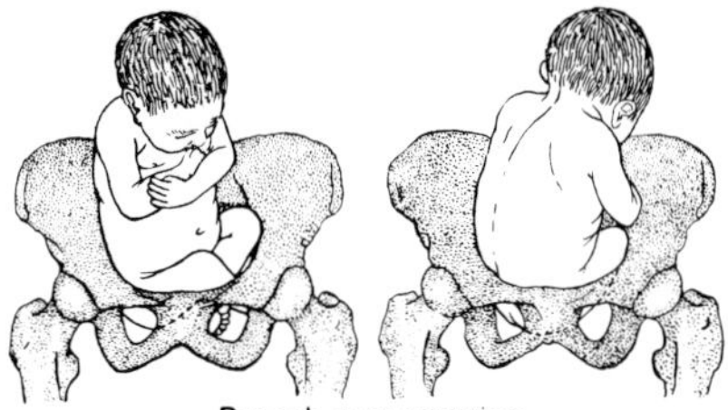

Breech presentation

Right sacroposterior — Right sacroanterior

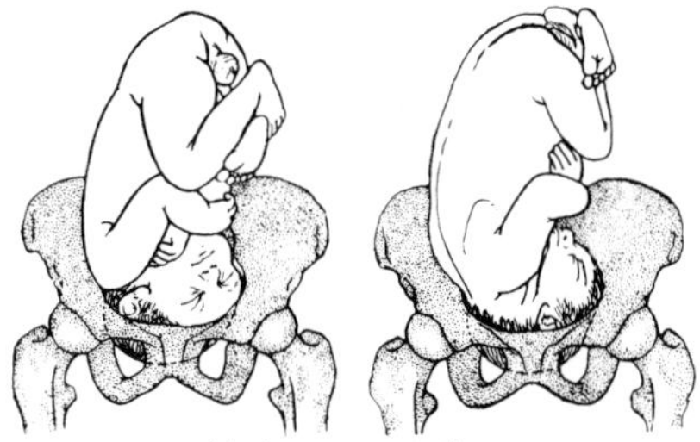

Vertex presentation

Right occipitoposterior — Right occipitoanterior

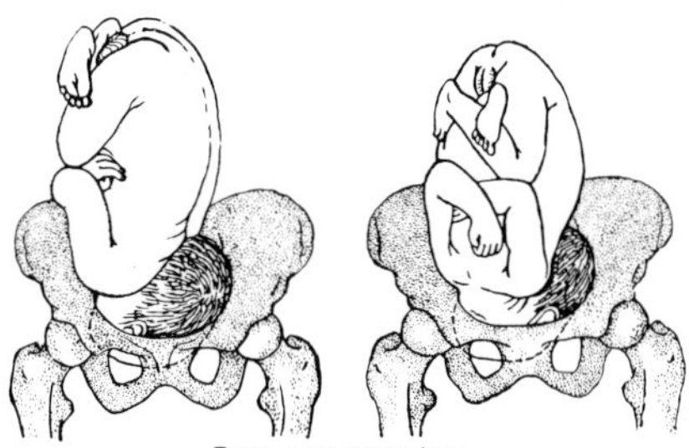

Face presentation

Right mentoposterior — Right mentoanterior

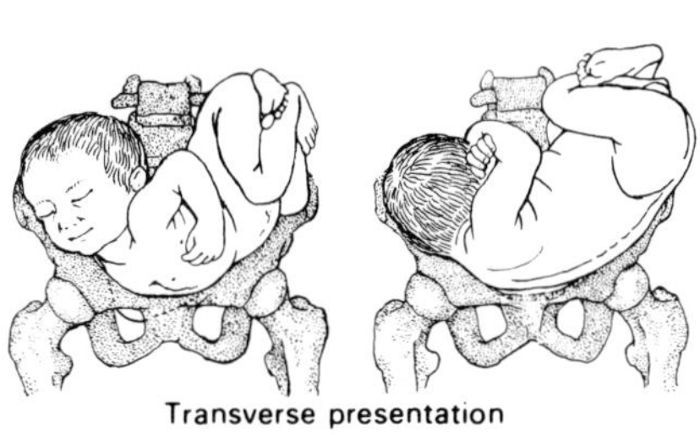

Transverse presentation

Right scapuloposterior — Right scapuloanterior

Presentations

No Lack of Talent

Giftedness comes in many forms. Academic talents make up only a small proportion of the sum total of abilities that deserve to be developed. Look over this list, and think about which strengths and abilities your child displays most strongly. Then let yourself be guided by your youngster's own interests, and provide materials or enrichment activities to draw out those talents.

- Acting ability
- Adventuresomeness
- Aesthetic perceptiveness
- Artistic talent
- Athletic prowess
- Common sense
- Compassion
- Courage
- Creativity
- Emotional maturity
- Excellent memory
- Imagination
- Inquiring mind
- Intuition
- Inventiveness
- Knowledge of a given subject
- Leadership abilities
- Literary aptitude
- Logical-reasoning ability
- Manual dexterity
- Mathematical ability
- Mechanical know-how
- Moral character
- Musicality
- Passionate interest in a specific topic
- Patience
- Persistence
- Physical coordination
- Political astuteness
- Problem-solving capacity
- Reflectiveness
- Resourcefulness
- Self-discipline
- Sense of humor
- Social savvy
- Spatial awareness
- Spiritual sensibility
- Strong will
- Verbal ability